POPULAR LOAN

This book is likely to be in heavy
demand. Please return on

Oxford Handbook of
Diabetes
Nursing

Oxford Handbooks in Nursing

Oxford Handbook of Midwifery
Janet Medforth, Susan Battersby, Maggie Evans, Beverley Marsh, and Angela Walker

Oxford Handbook of Mental Health Nursing
Edited by Patrick Callaghan and Helen Waldock

Oxford Handbook of Children's and Young People's Nursing
Edited by Edward Alan Glasper, Gillian McEwing, and Jim Richardson

Oxford Handbook of Nurse Prescribing
Sue Beckwith and Penny Franklin

Oxford Handbook of Cancer Nursing
Edited by Mike Tadman and Dave Roberts

Oxford Handbook of Cardiac Nursing
Edited by Kate Johnson and Karen Rawlings-Anderson

Oxford Handbook of Primary Care Nursing
Edited by Vari Drennan and Claire Goodman

Oxford Handbook of Gastrointestinal Nursing
Edited by Christine Norton, Julia Williams, Claire Taylor, Annmarie Nunwa, and Kathy Whayman

Oxford Handbook of Respiratory Nursing
Terry Robinson and Jane Scullion

Oxford Handbook of Nursing Older People
Beverley Tabernacle, Marie Barnes, and Annette Jinks

Oxford Handbook of Clinical Skills in Adult Nursing
Jacqueline Randle, Frank Coffey, and Martyn Bradbury

Oxford Handbook of Emergency Nursing
Robert Crouch, Alan Charters, Mary Dawood, and Paula O'Gara

Oxford Handbook of Dental Nursing
K Seymour, DYD Samarawickrama, EC Boon, and RL Parr

Oxford Handbook of Diabetes Nursing
Lorraine Avery and Sue Beckwith

Oxford Handbook of Musculoskeletal Nursing
Susan Oliver

Oxford Handbook of Women's Health Nursing
Ali Kubba, Sunanda Gupta, and Debra Holloway

Oxford Handbook of Perioperative Practice
Suzanne Hughes and Andy Mardell

Oxford Handbook of Critical Care Nursing
Sheila Adam and Sue Osborne

Oxford Handbook of Neuroscience Nursing
Sue Woodward, Cath Waterhouse

Oxford Handbook of General & Adult Nursing
Ann Close and George Castledine

Oxford Handbook of **Diabetes Nursing**

Edited by

Lorraine Avery

Medical Liaison Diabetes
Eli Lilly and Company Ltd
Hampshire, UK

and

Sue Beckwith

Doctoral Research Fellow
Consortium for Healthcare Research
Cornwall, UK

Editorial Advisor
Janet Sumner

Diabetes Specialist Nurse
Churchill Hospital
Oxford, UK

OXFORD
UNIVERSITY PRESS

OXFORD
UNIVERSITY PRESS

Great Clarendon Street, Oxford OX2 6DP

Oxford University Press is a department of the University of Oxford.
It furthers the University's objective of excellence in research, scholarship,
and education by publishing worldwide in

Oxford New York

Auckland Cape Town Dar es Salaam Hong Kong Karachi
Kuala Lumpur Madrid Melbourne Mexico City Nairobi
New Delhi Shanghai Taipei Toronto

With offices in

Argentina Austria Brazil Chile Czech Republic France Greece
Guatemala Hungary Italy Japan Poland Portugal Singapore
South Korea Switzerland Thailand Turkey Ukraine Vietnam

Oxford is a registered trade mark of Oxford University Press
in the UK and in certain other countries

Published in the United States
by Oxford University Press Inc., New York

British Library Cataloguing in Publication Data
Data available

Library of Congress Cataloging in Publication Data
Data available

Typeset by Cepha Imaging Private Ltd., Bangalore, India
Printed in
on acid-free paper by
Asia Pacific Offset

ISBN 978–0–19–954562–9

10 9 8 7 6 5 4 3 2 1

Preface

This pocket sized handbook aims to give an up-to-date, comprehensive and wherever possible evidence based, policy led and patient centred guidance to help all nurses who are caring for adults with diabetes.

The contents range from basic anatomy and physiology, through practical guidance on treatment and monitoring to policy and practice advice. References are given to aid the reader in supplementing the information given or to return to the source works.

The last chapter contains some fictitious case studies to contextualise and stimulate thought regarding treatment options.

We would like to express gratitude to our contributors for sharing their expertise with us. The contents have been peer and medically reviewed and we would like to thank our reviewers for their care and rigour.

Further we welcome constructive comments and recommendations from our readers and profoundly hope this handbook will help ensure safe and effective care delivery.

Lorraine Avery
Sue Beckwith

Foreword

The world of diabetes care is rapidly changing, not only in terms of the number of individuals affected by the condition and treatment options available, but also the location of care delivery.

The prevalence of diabetes in the United Kingdom has increased by over 1 million in the last decade, resulting in a total of 2.5 million people diagnosed with diabetes in 2008, of which approximately 90% have Type 2 diabetes. A significant proportion of health care professionals will come into contact with an individual with diabetes during each working day, a number of whom may not have any diabetes specific training, especially when you consider that 1 in every 10 patients occupying a hospital bed has diabetes.

The Diabetes National Service Framework (NSF) published in 2001 and 2003 and the introduction of the Quality and Outcome Framework (QOF) have had a significant impact on the way care is delivered, particularly to patients with Type 2 diabetes. Increasingly care is delivered in a primary care setting, improving access for many patients and expanding the number of healthcare professionals involved in diabetes care delivery.

As the number of individuals affected by diabetes expands so does the depth and breadth of evidence to support clinical practice. Rapid expansion in treatment options and combinations in recent years, together with the expansion in patient education provision and the promotion of patient participation in care planning and treatment decisions, presents an ongoing challenge for healthcare professionals to maintain up to date knowledge.

This book provides extensive information in a compact and portable format that will enable nurses and other health care professionals to readily access relevant evidence and information in a timely manner, whatever their area of clinical practice or level of experience. I am confident this book will be a valuable addition to the Oxford Handbook series, clinical libraries, and recommended reading lists for academic courses in diabetes.

Mags Bannister
Nurse Consultant in Diabetes
Chair RCN Diabetes Nurses Forum

23.2.09

Acknowledgements

I would like to thank everyone who has contributed to the development of this book, especially all of the chapter contributors listed on page xxi, and to Jan Sumner for her early inspiration.

Thanks also to the reviewers whose comments were constructive and contributed greatly to the final draft.

Finally I would like to thank my husband Chris for his never ending support during the journey of writing this book and my diabetes career.

Lorraine Avery

With acknowledgement to Jan Sumner for her help and inspiration from the inception to the completion of this handbook.

Thanks also goes to all those who have shared their knowledge with me and especially to those people with diabetes who have patiently taught me so much about what it is to live with this condition.

Sue Beckwith

Contents

Detailed contents

List of contributors

Susan Battersby
Independent Midwifery
Lecturer/Researcher
Sheffield, UK

Neil Baker
Senior Specialist Podiatrist
Ipswich Hospital
Ipswich, England

Philip Gardner
Diabetes Nurse Specialist
Bradford and Airedale Teaching
PCT
Bradford, UK

Beverley Marsh
Senior Midwifery Lecturer,
Sheffield Hallam University
Midwifery Practitioner, Sheffield
Teaching Hospitals Trust
Sheffield, UK

Beverley McDermott
Diabetes Nurse Specialist
Bradford and Airedale Teaching
PCT
Bradford, UK

Janet Medforth
Senior Lecturer
Faculty of Health and Well Being
Sheffield Hallam University
Sheffield, UK

Karen Prinsloo
Specialist Diabetes Dietician
Diabetes Centre, St Richard's
Hospital
Chichester, West Sussex, UK

Angela Walker
Senior Midwifery Lecturer and
Supervisor of Midwives
School of Nursing and Midwifery
University of Sheffield
Swinton, Rotherham, UK

Symbols and abbreviations

📖	cross-reference
<	less than
>	greater than
↑	increased
↓	decreased

A&E	Accident and Emergency
ACCORD	Action to Control Cardiovascular Risk in Diabetes
ACE	angiotensin-converting enzyme
ADA	American Diabetes Association
ARM	artificially ruptured membrane
bd	twice daily
BDI	Beck Depression Inventory
BG	blood glucose
BHS	British Hypertension Society
BMI	Body Mass Index
BNF	British National Formulary
bp	blood pressure
BR	background retinopathy
BSSM	British Society of Sexual Medicine
CABG	coronary artery bypass graft
CBA	controlled before and after studies
CF	counting fingers
CG	clinical governance
CHD	coronary heart disease
CHI	Commissioner for Health Improvement
CHO	carbohydrates
CPD	continuous professional development
CREST	Clinical Resources Efficiency Support Team
CSII	continuous subcutaneous infusion of insulin
CTG	cardiotocography
CV	cardiovascular
CVA	cerebrovascular accident
CVD	cardiovascular disease
DAFNE	Dose Adjustment for Normal Eating
DCCT	Diabetes Control and Complications Trial

DESMOND	Diabetes Education for Self-Management Ongoing and Newly Diagnosed
DKA	diabetic ketoacidosis
DM	diabetes mellitus
DoH	Department of Health
DPP	dipeptidyl peptidase
DPP-IV	dipeptidyl peptidase 4
DR	diabetic retinopathy
DUET	database of uncertainties about the effects of treatment
DVLA	Driver and Vehicle Licensing Authority
EAS	European Atherosclerosis Society
EASD	European Association Study for Diabetes
EBP	evidence-based practice
ECG	electrocardiogram
ED	erectile dysfunction
eGFR	estimated glomerula filtration rate
EHIC	European Health Insurance Card
ESR	erythrocyte sedimentation rate
FSH	follicle-stimulating hormone
GA	general anaesthesia
GAD	glutamic acid decarboxylase
GDM	gestational diabetes
GI	gastrointestinal
GIP	gastric inhibitory polypeptide
GII	glycaemic index
GLP1	glucagon-like peptide-1
GTN	glyceryl trinitrate
HAMD	Hamilton Rating Scale for Depression
HbA1c	haemoglobin A1c
HCP	health care professional
HDL	high density lipoprotein
HM	hand movement
HONK	hyperosmolar non-ketotic
HOT	hypertension optimal treatment
HPC	Health Professions Council
HPL	human placental lactogen
ICA	islet cell auto-antibodies
IDF	International Diabetes Foundation
IDL	intermediate density lipoprotein
IFG	impaired fasting *glucose*

IGT	impaired glucose tolerance
IHD	ischaemic heart disease
INR	international normalized ratio (blood coagulation)
IRMA	intraretinal microvascular abnormalities
IUD	intrauterine device
iv	intravenous
JDRF	Juvenile Diabetes Research Forum
LADA	latent autoimmune diabetes of adults
LDL	low density lipoprotein
LH	luteinizing hormone
LTC	long-term conditions
MDI	multiple daily injections
MDRD	modification of diet in renal disease
METS	metabolic equivalent of a task
MI	myocardial infarction
MODY	maturity Onset Diabetes of the Young
NELH	National Electronic Library for Health
NHS	National Health Service
NICE	National Institute for Health and Clinical Excellence
NLH	NHS electronic library for health
NMC	Nursing and Midwifery Council
NMF	nylon monofilament
NPC	National Prescribing Centre
NPfIT	National Programme for IT
NSC	National Screening Committee
NSF	National Service Framework
NVD	new vessels on disc
NVE	new vessels elsewhere
od	once daily
OGTT	oral glucose tolerance test
OTC	over the counter
PBC	practice-based commissioning
PCOS	polycystic ovary syndrome
PCT	Primary Care Trust
PDE5	phosphodiesterase type 5
PDP	personal development plans
PL	perception of light
POAD	peripheral obstructive arterial disease
PPR	pre-proliferative retinopathy

PVD	peripheral vascular disease
QOF	Quality and Outcomes Framework
QOL	quality of life
RCN	Royal College of Nursing
RCT	randomized controlled trials
RD&E	Royal Devon and Exeter Hospital
sc	subcutaneous
SEHD	Scottish Executive Health Department
SHA	strategic health authorities
SHEP	systolic hypertension in the elderly
SIGN	Scottish Intercollegiate Guidelines network
spyg	sphygmomanometer
STH	Sheffield Teaching Hospitals
TC	total cholesterol
tds	three times daily
TIA	transient ischaemic attack
U&E	urea and electrolytes
UKPDS	United Kingdom Prospective Diabetes Study
UTI	urinary tract infection
VA	visual acuity
VADT	Veterans Affairs Diabetes Trial
VDL	very low density lipoprotein
VEGF	vascular endothelial growth factor
VLDL	very low density lipoprotein
WAG	Welsh Assembly Government
WCC	white cell count
WHO	World Health Organization

Introduction

Background

Diabetes has existed as long as mankind. Hieroglyphs in the Egyptian pyramids and ancient Asian Sanskrit writings describe the symptoms only too familiar today (see 📖 Chapters 2 and 3).

Before the 1920s, when Banting and Best's discovered that insulin could be prepared and injected to alleviate the morbidity caused by Type 1 diabetes, the only treatment for this condition was a near starvation diet until the inevitability of death (Bliss 1982).

The National Service Framework (NSF) for Diabetes records the increase in numbers of people around the world who have been diagnosed with diabetes over the preceding decades. It is estimated that worldwide 246 million people have the disease (International Diabetes Federation 2007) and it is predicted that this will have doubled by the year 2010.

More than 2.5 million people in England have the disease with a disproportionate spread of those with Type 2 diabetes being of South Asian descent, and African and Afro-Caribbean origin (Qualities Outcome Framework 2007). Members of the poorest sectors of society fare the worst with increased risks of morbidity from complications of the disease.

It is estimated that more than half a million people in the UK have Type 2 diabetes without being aware of their condition and at least 50% already have some complications at the time of diagnosis (Diabetes UK, 2008). How to reach those at risk, but undiagnosed earlier is a problem that health practitioners need to have at the forefront of their minds.

Complications of diabetes are the leading causes of blindness in the working-age population, end-stage renal failure and, baring accidents, the greatest number of limb amputations.

Although the risk of developing Type 2 diabetes increases with age and obesity it can occur at any time, with recent significant increases in the numbers of those diagnosed with Maturity Onset Diabetes of the Young (MODY; see 📖 Classification of monogenetic diabetes, p. 14).

Further information

Bliss M. (1982) *The discovery of insulin*. University of Chicago Press, Chicago.

Department of Health (2001) *Diabetes National Service Framework*. Standards Stationery Office, London.

Diabetes UK (2008) Available at 🖥 http://diabetesuk.org (accessed 19 December 2008).

International Diabetes Federation (2007) *Diabetes Atlas 3rd Edition*. IDF: Brussels, Belgium.

Qualities Outcome Framework (2007) Available at 🖥 http://diabates.org.uk (accessed 19 December 2008).

The pancreas: overview

The pancreas is an elongated, leaf-shaped organ, pinkish in colour, lying across the back of the abdomen behind the stomach. The head of the pancreas, the widest part, lies to the right hand side in the curve of the first section of the small intestine, the duodenum.

The body of the pancreas, the tapered left-hand side, extends upwards towards the spleen, ending in the tail section. The pancreatic duct runs along the whole length of the pancreas.

The pancreas is covered with a thin connective tissue capsule that extends inward, partitioning the gland into lobules. It is made up of two types of cells – *exocrine* and *endocrine*. See Figure 1.1.

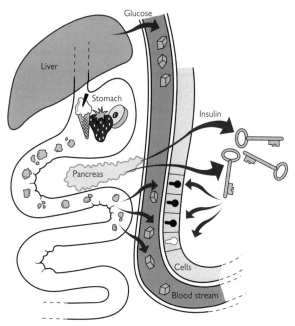

Fig. 1.1 Insulin action on the body. Insulin can be regarded as a key unlocking access to the cells. Reproduced from Matthews D et al (2008), *Diabetes*, with permission from Oxford University Press.

Exocrine functions of the pancreas

Exocrine anatomy

The majority of pancreatic cells are *exocrine cells* and their associated ducts. Embedded within this exocrine tissue are approximately 1 million grape-like cell clusters called acini. These are packed with membrane-bound secretory granules containing digestive enzymes, which pass through larger and larger ducts until they flow into the main pancreatic duct and drain into the duodenum.

Exocrine physiology

Secretions from the exocrine cells are vital to enable food to be completely digested:
- As chyme, the bolus of partially digested food, enters the small intestine it is acidic and needs to be *neutralized* to protect the duodenal mucosa.
- Proteins, fats and starch need to be further broken down before they can be absorbed into the blood stream.

Secretion of bicarbonate (a base) and water:
- Secreted from the endothelia cells that line the pancreatic duct.
- Vital for neutralizing the acidity of the chyme.

Protein digestion

- Facilitated by the two major pancreatic proteases, trypsin and chymotrypsin.
- Proteases are synthesized and packaged into secretory vesicles as the proenzymes trypsinogen and chymotrypsinogen.
- Inactive as proenzymes to preserve protein of the pancreatic cells.

Fat digestion

- Triglyceride, or neutral lipid, cannot be directly absorbed across the intestinal mucosa.
- First digested into a 2-monoglyceride and two free fatty acids.
- Pancreatic lipase performs this hydrolysis, delivered into the duodenum as a constituent of pancreatic juice.

Starch digestion

- Amylase (technically alpha-amylase) is the enzyme that hydrolyses starch to maltose.
- The major source of amylase is pancreatic secretions, although amylase is also present in saliva.

In addition, the pancreas produces other digestive enzymes including:
- Ribonuclease.
- Deoxyribonuclease.
- Gelatinase.
- Elastase.

Endocrine functions of the pancreas

Endocrine anatomy

Humans have approximately 1 million *endocrine* cells, called the *Islets of Langerhans*, which comprise five cell types.

Three major cell types are:
• Alpha cells, which secrete *glucagon*.
• Beta cells, which produce *insulin*.
• Delta cells, which secrete the hormone *somatostatin* (also produced by other endocrine cells).

The central part of each islet is occupied by beta cells, and the alpha and delta cells cover this hub.

The Islets have a very good vascular supply receiving 10–15% of the pancreatic blood flow, although they make up only 1–2% of the total pancreatic mass. The pancreas is served by the:
• Gastro-duodenal arteries.
• Branches of the splenic artery.
• The splenic vein and artery run superiorly and posteriorly.
• The mesenteric vein lies in the angle between the head and body of the pancreas.

This facilitates secreted hormones to pass readily into the general circulation.

The secretion of insulin and glucagon are controlled by both parasympathetic and sympathetic neurons.

Endocrine physiology

The three hormones secreted by the endocrine tissue in the pancreas regulate the levels of glucose in the blood. They are:
• **Insulin**, which lowers blood glucose (BG) levels.
• **Glucagon**, which promotes the release of glycogen from the liver, raising BG levels.
• **Somatostatin**, which prevents the release of the other two hormones.

Insulin and glucagon are critical participants in glucose homeostasis and serve as acute regulators of blood glucose concentration (see Fig. 1.2).

Insulin is enormously important – a deficiency in insulin or deficits in insulin responsiveness lead to diabetes mellitus.

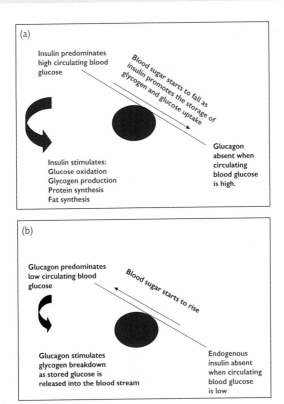

Fig. 1.2 Blood glucose regulation. (a) Fed state post-prandial. (b) Fasting state pre-prandial or after having missed a meal.

Hormones

Insulin

A small protein composed of two peptide chains, A and B chains:
- The A chain consists of 21 amino acids.
- The B chain of 30 amino acids.
- Synthesized in significant quantities only in B cells in the pancreas.

Glucagon

This is the counter regulatory hormone to insulin:
- A linear peptide of 29 amino acids.
- Synthesized as proglucagon within the alpha cells of the pancreas.
- Secreted in response to:
  • hypoglycaemia;
  • elevated blood levels of amino acids;
  • exercise (it is not clear whether it is exercise *per se* or the accompanying exercise-induced depletion of glucose).

When BG levels fall, glucagon is secreted. It facilitates the rise in BG levels in two ways:
- Glucagon stimulates breakdown of glycogen stored in the liver.
- Glucagon activates hepatic gluconeogenesis (production of glucose). Gluconeogenesis is the pathway by which non-hexose substrates, such as amino acids are converted to glucose.

Glucagon also appears to have a minor effect of enhancing lipolysis of tri-glyceride in adipose tissue, which could be viewed as an additional means of conserving blood glucose by providing fatty acid fuel to most cells.

Somatostatin

This was first discovered in hypothalamic extracts and identified as a hormone that inhibited secretion of growth hormone. Subsequently, somatostatin was found to be secreted by a broad range of tissues including:
- Pancreas.
- Intestinal tract.
- Central nervous system (outside the hypothalamus).

Effects on the pancreas
- Inhibits secretion of insulin and glucagon.
- Suppresses pancreatic exocrine secretions.

Diabetes: an overview

Definition

Diabetes is a group of metabolic conditions, which are chronic and progressive, and are all characterized by an elevated blood glucose level. It impacts on almost every aspect of life, and affects the psychological and physiological well being of those who have been diagnosed with the condition.

Chronic hyperglycaemia causes damage to the eyes, kidneys, heart, blood vessels, and nervous tissue.

Current classification

The World Health Organization (WHO) reclassified diabetes in 1999 when the terms Type 1 and Type 2 diabetes were reintroduced.

The classification of diabetes is based on the underlying cause (Table 1.1) within the categories Type 1, Type 2 gestational diabetes, and other types.

Type 1

This is an autoimmune disease resulting from islet β cell destruction and is associated with:
- Pancreatic islet cell deficiency.
- Anti-glutamic acid decarboxylase (GAD) antibodies.
- Islet cell antibodies.
- Insulin antibodies.

People with Type 1 diabetes are prone to ketoacidosis (see 📖 Diabetic ketoacidosis, p. 172).

Type 2

This comprises between 75 and 95% of all cases of diabetes, and is classified with defective insulin secretion or action.

It is associated with:
- Insulin resistance.
- Insulin secretion deficit.
- Or a combination of both.

Further information

Expert Committee on the Diagnosis and Classification of Diabetes Mellitus. (2003) Report of the expert committee on the diagnosis and classification of diabetes mellitus. *Diabetes Care* **26**, S5–20.

Table 1.1 Diabetes Types 1 and 2 compared

	Type 1	Type 2
Phenotype	Onset mainly in childhood and adolescence	Onset mainly after 40 years of age; however, increase in numbers of cases in the young
	95% develop the disease before the age of 25	Risks rise steeply with age. 1 in 20 of those over 65 years have Type 2 diabetes. 1 in 5 of those over 85 years of age
	Often thin or unintentionally losing weight.	Often obese
	Ketoacidosis often a presenting feature	Not prone to ketoacidosis
	Absolute insufficiency of insulin, therefore requires insulin replacement to survive	Relative insufficiency of insulin or insulin resistance, therefore does not need insulin replacement to survive
	Pancreatic damage caused by an autoimmune attack	No autoimmune attack on the pancreas
Treatment	Insulin injections are essential treatment, alongside healthy diet and exercise	Staged approach: 1 Healthy diet 2 Regular exercise 3 Weight loss if indicated 4 Hypoglycaemic/anti-diabetic medication 5 Insulin injections
Genotype	Increased prevalence in relatives	Increased prevalence in relatives
	Identical twin study >50% concordance	Identical twin study above 70% concordance
	Equal presentation men and women	More women, especially those who have had gestational diabetes. Increase prevalence in those of South Asian, African, African Caribbean, Hispanic, and Middle Eastern decent

Classification of monogenetic diabetes

Diabetes caused by inherited monogenetic defects in beta cell function, previously called maturity onset diabetes of the young (MODY), is found mainly in those under 25 years of age. It is characterized by mild hyperglycaemia. In contrast to Type 2 diabetes, insulin action remains unimpaired, but insulin secretion is reduced. Inheritance follows an autosomal dominant pattern which means a parent with MODY has a 50% chance of passing it on to their offspring (autosomals are one of the 22 non-sexually specific chromosomes).

Each type of MODY is caused by a single gene not working properly (monogenetic). The first MODY gene was identified in 1992 (Hattersley et al 1992), and there are more than 6 known genes, each causing a different form of monogenetic diabetes (Fajans et al 2001). The defective genes are responsible for the body's glucose sensor (glucokinase) and factors that control the production of insulin in the beta cells of the Islets of Langerhans in the pancreas (HNF-1alpha, HNF-1beta, HNF-4alpha, IPF-1, and NEURO-D1).

The different types of MODY make up between 2 and 5% of the population of people who have diabetes, but who do have endogenous insulin. MODY X refers to those where a particular genetic mutation has not yet been identified.

HNF-4alpha or HNF-4a (MODY 1)

This rare type is caused by a mutation of the *HNF-4* gene on chromosome 20q and has an effect similar to MODY3.

Glucokinase (MODY 2)

- Causes between 10 and 65% of MODY.
- Causes mild diabetes that rarely leads to complications.
- Often treated with meal planning and diet alone.
- Often diagnosed in childhood or pregnancy.

HNF-1alpha or HNF-1a (MODY 3)

Caused by mutations on chromosome 12, HNF-1alpha is the most commonly found MODY (WHO 1999).

- Causes between 20 and 75% of MODY.
- Causes progressive diabetes.
- Potential for complications of diabetes to develop.
- Usually diagnosed after puberty.
- Sensitive to sulphonylureas.

IPF-1 (MODY 4)

Rare form of MODY producing relatively mild diabetes.

HNF-1beta (MODY 5)

Rare form of MODY associated with kidney disease.

Further information

Fajans S, Bell G, Polonsky K. (2001) Molecular mechanisms and clinical pathophysiology of Maturity Onset Diabetes of the Young. *N Engl J Med* **345**, 971.

Hattersley AT, Turner RC, Permutt MA, et al (1992) Linkage of Type 2 diabetes to the glucokinase gene. *Lancet* **339**(8805), 1307–10.

World Health Organization (1999) *Definition, diagnosis and classification of diabetes mellitus and its complications: report of a WHO consultation. Part 1: diagnosis and classification of diabetes mellitus.* Geneva: World Health Organization.

Genetic testing

It is estimated that 1% of people with diabetes in the UK (about 20,000 people) have monogenetic diabetes (Shepherd 2001).

The Royal Devon and Exeter Hospital (RD&E) has funding for a project that delivers further training regarding monogenetic diabetes and genetic testing to 18 experienced diabetes specialist nurses. Each nurse will be based in a different region of the UK and will offer:

• Updating to local diabetes teams regarding monogenetic diabetes and the genetic tests available.
• Assistance identifying which families are likely to have monogenic diabetes.
• Advice regarding the most appropriate diagnostic genetic test to use.

They can also discuss implications with the families and guide follow-up for the family members once the results are received.

Predictive testing

It is possible to test individuals who have a parent with MODY to see if they have inherited the impaired gene, and this is called predictive testing.

• If a parent has MODY then there is a 50% (1:2) chance that their offspring will have the same the gene and will go on to develop diabetes.
• A predictive genetic test looks at the genetic code to see if the same genetic changes are present.
• A venous blood sample is sent to the RD&E for examination.
• Results either positive or negative are available in 4–8 weeks:
  • *positive* – the person is likely to develop diabetes at some time in the future and regular blood glucose checks should be undertaken;
  • *negative* – the risk factors for developing diabetes are the same as for the rest of the population.

Why test?
• If a differential diagnosis is made this will lead to the provision of optimal treatment.
• Mistakes can be made by teams who do not have the experience or latest information regarding the implications of the different types of MODY, for example:
  • people with HNF-1alpha (MODY 3) are sensitive to sulphonylureas and often achieve better glycaemic control on a small dose of these compared with insulin injections.
  • mutations within the glucokinase gene (MODY 2) cause mild, stable hyperglycaemia, which does not require treatment, but in children may be misdiagnosed as Type 1 diabetes.

Further information

Shepherd M. (2001) Recognising maturity onset diabetes of the young. *J Diabetes Nurs* **5**(6), 168–72.
Shepherd M, Sparkes AC, Hattersley AT. (2001) Genetic testing in Maturity Onset Diabetes of the Young (MODY): a new challenge for the diabetes clinic. *Pract Diabetes Internat* **18**, 16–21.

Disease-related diabetes

Diseases of exocrine function
- Pancreatitis.
- Pancreatectomy following trauma or surgery.
- Neoplasia.
- Pancreatic destruction, for example, with cystic fibrosis.
- Fibrocalculous pancreatopathy.
- Haemochromatosis (a disease of iron storage).

Diseases of the endocrine system

Cushing's syndrome
- Increases the production of glucose by the liver.
- Increases insulin resistance at the peripheral tissue level.
- Resulting in increased blood glucose.

Acromegaly
- Usually caused by a tumour in the pituitary gland, which causes excess growth hormone to be produced.
- Growth hormone increases insulin resistance.
- Over half of patients with acromegaly have hyperinsulinemia and glucose intolerance.

Pheochromocytoma
- Excess epinephrine, a 'fight or flight' hormone is secreted, often because of a phenochromocytoma, a tumour of the adrenal gland.
- Fight or flight response mobilizes glucose production in order to fuel the activity.
- Epinephrine acts on adrenoreceptors and increases insulin resistance.
- Inhibits insulin secretion and increases the breakdown of fat and glycogen to glucose in the liver.
- This can result in diabetes.

Glucagonoma
Rare tumours of the pancreatic alpha cells may increase glucagons levels resulting in impaired glucose regulation.

Somatostatinoma
- Excess somastatin secretion caused by a rare pancreatic tumour affecting the pancreatic delta cells.
- Inhibits insulin secretion and results in impaired glucose regulation.

Drug and chemical interactions

Many medications prescribed for specific purposes can inhibit the effect of insulin, not causing diabetes, but acting as a trigger in those with a predisposition to develop it.

Some hormones when given in large doses can impair the action of insulin, e.g. glucocorticoids and thyroid hormones.

It is important to check the current edition of the British National Formulary (BNF) for full details of drug interactions and contra-indications.

Patients who need to take contraindicated medications will need to be aware of the additional risks of hyperglycaemia. Appropriate monitoring is required in order to be able to react to unsafe blood glucose levels.

Glucocorticoids
- Raise blood glucose levels by counteracting some actions of insulin.
- Prolonged use of prednisolone may lead to glucose intolerance and diabetes.

Thiazides (diuretics)
- Can increase hyperglycaemia in people with Type 2 diabetes.
- Impairing insulin secretion as a result of causing potassium depletion.
- May also increase insulin resistance.

Gestational diabetes

Gestational diabetes (diabetes in pregnancy) affects less than 1 in 20 women.

It is thought that placental hormones increase insulin resistance in the mother leading to elevated blood glucose levels.

- Usually identified in the second trimester.
- If hyperglycaemia persists requires treatment with insulin for the duration of the pregnancy.
- Blood glucose levels return to normal following delivery.
- Usually occurs in subsequent pregnancies.
- Can often be an indicator of Type 2 diabetes in later life (see 📖 Chapter 2, pp. 27–52).
- Severe insulin resistance with circulating antibodies to the insulin receptor is known as Type B insulin resistance.
- Hyperglycaemia can be caused when anti-insulin receptor antibodies bind to the insulin receptor, blocking insulin from its receptors.
- Rarely these autoantibodies can cause hypoglycaemia by mimicking the action of insulin.

Impaired-fasting glucose

Those who have fasting blood glucose above the normal range (less than 6.1mmol/l), but below the diagnostic range for diabetes (greater then 7mmol/l).

A study in Helsinki (Qiao et al 2003) of 2593 people over 10 years showed the risk of progression to diabetes was 1 in 50 for an adult aged 45–64 years with normal fasting glucose, but rose to 1 in 22 for an adult with impaired fasting glucose.

Men and women had the same level of risk.

Further information

Qiao Q, Lindström J, Valle T, Tuomilehto J (2003). Progression to clinically diagnosed and treated diabetes from impaired glucose tolerance and impaired fasting glycaemia. *Diabetes Med* **20**, 1027–33.

Diagnosis and diagnostic criteria

Diabetes mellitus

WHO (2006) does not discriminate between Types 1 and 2, identifying people with diabetes as 'a group with significantly increased premature mortality and increased risk of microvascular and cardiovascular complications', and the diagnostic criteria for this group as having:

- A fasting plasma glucose ≥ 7.0mmol/l (126mg/dl).
- Or a 2h plasma glucose ≥ 11.1mmol/l (200mg/dl).

Type 1 (see Table 1.2)

- If classical symptoms present, confirm diagnosis by a single laboratory glucose measurement.
- If classical symptoms not present, confirm diagnosis by two laboratory glucose measurements (NICE 2004).

Diagnosis of diabetes mellitus is made if there are positive tests from any two of the following on different days:

- Symptoms of diabetes mellitus plus random blood glucose concentration above 11mmol/l.[1]

or

- Fasting plasma glucose above 7.00mmol/l.

or

- 2h post-prandial blood glucose above 11.1mmol/l following a 75g glucose load (a glucose tolerance test).

Type 2 (see Table 1.3)

The National Collaborating Centre for Chronic Conditions updated the NICE National Clinical Guidelines NICE in 2008 describing people with Type 2 diabetes as:

> People are normally thought to have Type 2 diabetes if they do not have Type 1 diabetes (rapid onset, often in childhood, insulin-dependent, ketoacidosis if neglected) or other medical conditions or treatment suggestive of secondary diabetes. (NICE 2008)

Gestational diabetes

A standard oral glucose tolerance test should be performed. The World Health Organization (WHO) recommends:

- Overnight (8–14h) fasting.
- 75g anhydrous glucose in 200–300ml water.
- Measure plasma glucose fasting and 2h after the glucose loading.
- A diagnosis is made if the fasting blood glucose is above 5.3mmol/l and the 2h post-glucose load is above 8.6mmol/l.

(see 📖 Gestational diabetes, p. 19).

---

1 Symptoms include polydipsia, polyurea, recurrent infections, or unexplained or unintended weight loss.

Table 1.2 Signs and symptoms of Type 1 diabetes

Initial signs and symptoms	Reason
Rarely diabetic ketoacidosis (DKA)	It is unusual for patients to present with ketoacidosis unless precipitated by trauma, infection, or surgery
Polyuria (frequently passing urine)	Caused by osmotic diuresis secondary to hyperglycaemia
Polydipsia (thirst)	Caused by the hyperosmolar state and dehydration caused by polyurea
Polyphagia with weight loss	Weight loss with a normal or increased appetite is due to depletion of water, and a catabolic state with reduced glycogen, proteins, and triglycerides
Fatigue and weakness	Due to muscle wasting from the catabolic state of insulin deficiency, hypovolemia[1], and hypokalemia[2]
Muscle cramps	Due to electrolyte imbalance
Blurred vision	Due to the effect of the hyperosmolar state on the lens and vitreous humor. Glucose and its metabolites cause dilation of the lens, altering its normal focal length
Gastrointestinal symptoms: • Nausea • Abdominal discomfort or pain • Changes in bowel habit	Acute fatty liver may lead to distention of the hepatic capsule, causing right upper quadrant pain. Pancreatitis may cause abdominal pain. Abdominal pain often accompanies ketosis.

[1]Hypovolemia: decrease in blood plasma volume.

[2]Hypokalemia: decreased blood potassium levels.

Table 1.3 Diagnostic criteria Type 2, IGT, IFG

Plasma glucose (mmol/l)	Fasting plasma glucose	2h post-glucose tolerance test
Diabetes mellitus	≥7.00	≥11.1
Impaired glucose tolerance (IGT)	>7.00	Between 7.8 and 11
Impaired fasting glucose (IFG)	6.1–7	>7.8
Non-diabetic response	6.1	7.75

NB. In the absence of symptoms, diabetes should only be diagnosed on the basis of two abnormal glucose results. One abnormal result is sufficient if the patient has symptoms.

Further information

WHO (1999). *Definition, Diagnosis and Classification of Diabetes Mellitus and its Complications.* World Health Organization, Geneva.

http://www.staff.ncl.ac.uk/philip.home/who_dmc.htm#Diagnosis (accessed 24 November 2007).

National Institute for Clinical Excellence (NICE) (2004) *Type 1 diabetes: diagnosis and management of type 1 diabetes in adults.* NICE, London.

WHO (2006) *Definition and diagnosis of diabetes mellitus and intermediate hyperglycaemia.* World Health Organization, Geneva.

Differential diagnosis

This is the (often mental) checklist of hypothesized alternative diagnoses made in response to a patient's symptoms, history, appearance, and clinical parameters. For example, if a patient has glycosuria (glucose in their urine), it is important to consider the following possible causes.

Endocrine disorders

- **Endocrine tumour** causing increased production of growth hormone:
  - glucocorticoids
  - catecholamines
  - glucagon
  - somatostatin.
- **Addison disease.**
- **Graves disease.**
- **Hashimoto thyroiditis.**
- **Acanthosis nigricans** (genetic disorders with insulin resistance).

Drugs

- Thiazides.
- Diuretics.
- Phenytoin.
- Glucocorticoids.

Chronic pancreatitis

Cystic fibrosis

Prader–Willi syndrome

- Mental retardation.
- Muscular hypotonia (low muscle tone, and reduced muscle strength).
- Obesity.
- Short stature.
- Hypogonadism (lack of function of the ovaries or testes associated with diabetes mellitus (DM)).

Renal glycosuria

Glucose appears in urine despite normal glucose concentration in blood. This glucose may be due to:
- An autosomal genetic disorder.
- Dysfunction of the proximal renal tubule (e.g. Fanconi syndrome, chronic renal failure).
- Increased glucose load on tubules by the elevated glucose filtration rate during pregnancy.

Peripheral neuropathy

- Due to alcohol and vitamin B12 deficiency.

Chapter 2

Type 2 diabetes

Incidence and epidemiology

Type 2 diabetes is the most common form of diabetes accounting for approximately 85–95% of all diagnosed diabetes. The World Health Organization (WHO) has predicted that by 2025 the global prevalence will reach 300 million. The increase in the prevalence of Type 2 diabetes is closely associated with the rise in obesity. The rise in obesity rates parallels that in Type 2 diabetes. This has been correlated with the reduction of physical activity and the higher consumption of calorie dense foods.

Ethnicity

The prevalence of Type 2 diabetes varies more than 10-fold between the highest and lowest risk populations. The lowest prevalence (<3%) in less developed countries, the highest prevalence 30–50% of adults in, for example, North American Indians, South Asians, and Aborigines (Krentz & Bailey 2007).

Ethnicity is an important risk factor for the development of insulin resistance and central obesity.

Family history

Type 2 diabetes is associated with a family history of the condition. The risk associated with developing diabetes if a parent has it is approximately 40%, rising to 50% if both parents have Type 2 diabetes. Identical twins have a 90% concordance of developing Type 2 diabetes; this strongly supports the genetic component as a risk factor for developing Type 2 diabetes.

Age

The incidence of diabetes increases with age. It is recognized that glucose tolerance decreases with age, and this has been associated with weight gain and reduced physical activity in this group. It is not clear whether age *per se* leads to a lack of insulin production and reduced sensitivity to insulin as part of the ageing process occurs.

Foetal gene hypothesis

In population studies, low birth weight has been correlated with an increased risk for the development of Type 2 diabetes in middle age. The risk becomes greater if obesity develops in adulthood. It has been suggested that intrauterine malnutrition leads to less beta cells and insulin resistance.

Gender

The prevalence of Type 2 diabetes in both males and females is equivalent, although post-menopausal women with multi-pregnancies appear to have a greater risk of developing Type 2 diabetes as do women who have had previous gestational diabetes.

Further information

Krentz AJ & Bailey CJ (2007). *Type 2 diabetes in practice*. The Royal Society of Medicine Press Ltd., London.

Aetiology

Type 2 diabetes is associated with defects in insulin secretion and the action of insulin. The reduction in sensitivity to insulin (insulin resistance) precedes the decrease in insulin production; insulin resistance is a primary defect, 92% of patients with Type 2 diabetes will be insulin resistant. (Haffner 1999). At the time of diagnosis, beta cell function and the production of insulin are reduced by 50% and this continues to decline as Type 2 diabetes progresses (see Fig. 2.1).

Insulin resistance

This is associated with a group of clinical features known as the metabolic syndrome (see Fig. 2.2).

Insulin resistance precedes the diagnosis of diabetes. As the bodies' ability to effectively utilize the insulin is reduced, hyperglycaemia occurs.

Hyperinsulinaemia

As insulin resistance develops and increases with the duration of diabetes, the immediate response of beta cells is to increase production of insulin; this is known as hyperinsulinaemia. Beta cell over-work eventually leads to beta cell failure and reduced production of insulin. At diagnosis, 50% of beta cells are failing to produce any insulin, which decreases at approximately 4% per year.

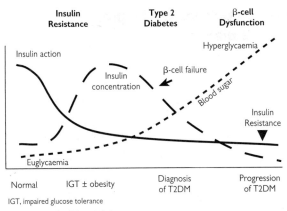

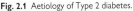

IGT, impaired glucose tolerance

Fig. 2.1 Aetiology of Type 2 diabetes.

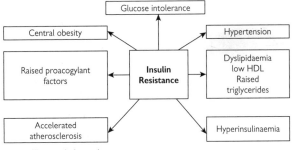

Fig. 2.2 The metabolic syndrome.

Further information

Haffner SM, D'Agostino R Jr, Mykkänen L et al (1999). Insulin sensitivity in subjects with type 2 diabetes. Relationship to cardiovascular risk factors: the Insulin Resistance Atherosclerosis Study. *Diabetes Care* **22**, 562–8.

Risk factors for developing Type 2 diabetes

- Obesity, high waist circumference.
- Family history.
- Ethnicity.
- Age.
- Lifestyle issues, e.g. reduced physical activity and smoking.
- Previous history of gestational diabetes.
- Impaired fasting glycaemia or impaired glucose tolerance.
- Other endocrine disorders, thyrotoxicosis, Cushings syndrome, acrogmegaly.
- Hyperglycaemic drugs, e.g. steroids and some anti-psychotics.
- Low birth weight.
- Schizophrenia and severe mental illness.

Further information

Bushe C, Holt R. (2004) Diabetes prevalence in schizophrenia. *Br J Psychiat* **184** (Suppl 47), 67–71.

Presentation

Type 2 diabetes usually presents in middle age or later life. However, increasingly Type 2 diabetes is presenting in younger age groups, including children. The onset is usually insidious and may go undiagnosed for a number of years. Increasingly people are being diagnosed as a result of routine screening in cardiovascular clinics. Commonly, patients present without the classical symptoms of hyperglycaemia, although recurrent fungal infections may precede diagnosis.

Type 2 diabetes may also present as hyperosmolar non-ketotic coma (HONK; see 📖 p. 174).

Clinical features of Type 2 diabetes

- Usually >45 years of age.
- Obesity >75% of cases.
- Symptoms of hyperglycaemia, absent, or mild.
- Ketone negative.
- Insulin resistance.
- Relative insulin deficiency.
- Metabolic syndrome often present.
- Progressive in nature, requiring increasing therapeutic intervention.
- Increased risk of macrovascular complications.

Principles of treatment

Aims of treatment

- To achieve blood glucose levels, bp, and lipid profiles to target levels according to national and international guidelines.
- Reduce weight and waist circumference in most cases.
- Relief of symptoms.
- Reduce risk of micro- and macrovascular complications.
- Decrease mortality from cardiovascular disease.
- Maintain quality of life.

Targets in Type 2 diabetes (NICE 2008)

HbA1c	6.5%
Fasting plasma glucose	<7.0mmol/l
Post meal glucose	<8.5mmol/l
Blood pressure	<130/80 if renal, eye, or cerebrovascular complications are present
Blood pressure	<140/80 in the absence of above complications
Total cholesterol	<4.0mmol/l
HDL cholesterol	>1.1mmol/l
LDL cholesterol	<2.0mmol/l

Management guidelines

The management guidelines produced by the American Diabetes Association (ADA) and the European Association Study for Diabetes (EASD) recommend that all patients are provided with diet and lifestyle advice, and metformin is commenced at diagnosis. The second line agent will depend on a number of factors. The aim of treatment as suggested in the guidelines is to treat an HbA1c above 7.0%. See Fig 2.3.

Management of hyperglycemia in type 2 diabetes

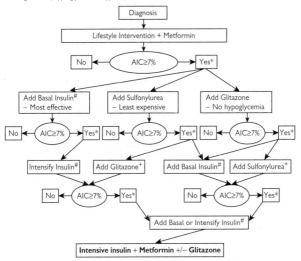

Fig. 2.3 Simplified ADA/EASD consensus algorithm for Type 2 diabetes (Nathan et al 2006).

Further information

Nathan DM, Buse JB, Davidson MB et al (2006). Management of hyperglycemia in type 2 diabetes: A consensus algorithm for the initiation and adjustment of therapy: a consensus statement from the American Diabetes Association and the European Association for the Study of Diabetes. *Diabetes Care* **29**(8), 1963–72.

NICE (2008). *Type 2 diabetes: the management of type 2 diabetes*. NICE, London. ☐ http://www.nice.org.uk/CG66

Diet and lifestyle intervention

The majority of people presenting with Type 2 diabetes are overweight. The UKPDS demonstrated only 16% of newly diagnosed Type 2's achieved a target HA1c after 3 months on diet alone. Alongside this it was demonstrated the higher the fasting glucose at diagnosis the less likely Type 2 patients are to achieve good control on diet alone.

A dietary assessment is essential to establish current eating habits with the aim of achieving current dietary recommendations.

Principles of dietary management of Type 2 diabetes

- Regular meals, to include a moderate portion of starchy carbohydrate at each meal.
- Maintaining a varied diet including food choices from all food groups – carbohydrates, protein, and fat.
- Aiming for 5 portions of fruit and vegetables a day.
- ↓ Intake of sucrose and refined carbohydrate foods in line with general healthy eating.
- Encouraging more low glycaemic index (GI) food choices.
- ↓ Total fat intake – reduction especially of saturated fat whilst encouraging monounsaturated fats.
- ↓ Salt intake.
- Alcohol in moderation.
- Aiming for a healthy weight or maintaining weight.
- Avoid 'diabetic food' products.

(See 📖 Chapter 4, pp. 69–80.)

Unfortunately, dietary management of Type 2 diabetes to achieve long-term good control tends too be short-lived, as adherence to dietary recommendations is generally poor. The progression of Type 2 diabetes will mean the majority of patients will require poly-pharmacy within a few years of diagnosis.

Previous recommendations suggested, at diagnosis, a 3 month period on diet alone. This has now been replaced by the joint ADA and EASD Group consensus guidelines, which recommend the early introduction of metformin at diagnosis (see Fig. 2.3).

Exercise

Exercise is an integral part of the management of Type 2 diabetes. Physical activity (particularly if it is aerobic) improves:
- Insulin sensitivity.
- Blood glucose control.
- Increases HDL.
- Facilitates weight loss.
- Improves cardiovascular health.
- Can have a positive impact on mood, and help relieve depression and stress.

Current recommendations suggest 30min of moderate activity on at least 5 days per week. Moderate activity is defined as any activity that leaves the individual slightly breathless, but still able to talk whilst undertaking the activity.

Structured education

NICE Guidelines (2008) recommend that structured education is offered to all newly-diagnosed people with Type 2 diabetes and annually thereafter to reinforce information provided.

It is essential that health care professionals are aware of programmes available locally and ensure these are integrated with care pathways. See Structured education: meeting NICE criteria, p.106.

Metformin

First line therapy in all patients with Type 2 diabetes.

Mode of action
- Reduces hepatic glucose production (gluconeogenesis).
- Reduces glucose absorption at gut level.
- Improves insulin sensitivity, although the actual mechanism of this is unclear.

Side effects
Gastrointestinal side effects, abdominal distension, abdominal pain, metallic taste in mouth, loss of appetite, nausea, diarrhoea.

Benefits
- Does not cause weight gain and, in some cases, may facilitate weight loss.
- In the UKPDS, metformin showed a greater effect on any diabetes-related end point. All cause mortality and stroke.

Starting doses should initially be low to facilitate tolerance
Starting dose would typically be 500 or 850mg once daily, titrating to maximum tolerated doses.

In clinical practice the dose is rarely taken above 2550mg, e.g. 850mg tds. The majority of clinicians use 1g bd as the maximum dose (see Table 2.1).

Contraindications
Metformin should be avoided for those patients with:
- Renal failure (eGFR < 30, and/or creatinine > 130mmol/l.
- Hepatic failure.
- Significant cardiac or respiratory failure.

The risk of lactic acidosis, which is a rare, but serious side effect that carries a high mortality, is greater in patients with the above contraindications.

See BNF for full prescribing information.

Table 2.1 Some examples of metformin doses and range

Name	Initial dose	Maximum dose
Metformin	500–850mg	2g
Metformin SR	500mg	2g
Metformin SR	750mg	1.5g

Sulphonylureas and post-prandial regulators

Rarely used as a first line therapy, unless presenting glucose is high and the patient is symptomatic of hyperglycaemia, losing weight and the individual is not obese.

Mode of action
- Stimulate insulin secretion by binding to sulphonylurea receptors on the beta cell membrane.
- Require preserved beta cell function to achieve the above.
- Post-prandial regulators have a similar mode of action to sulphonlyureas (binding on different receptor site in the beta cell) the onset of action tends to be faster and has a shorter duration of action.

Side effects
- Hypoglycaemia.
- Weight gain.
- Occasional skin reactions (rash).

Contraindications
- Pregnancy and breast feeding.
- Ketoacidosis.
- Renal and hepatic impairment.

(See Tables 2.2 and 2.3. See BNF for full prescribing information.)

Table 2.2 Some examples of sulphonylureas doses and range

Name	Initial dose	Maximum dose
Glicazide	40–80mg	320mg (160mg bd)
Gliclazide MR	30mg	120mg od
Glipizide	2.5–5mg	20mg
Glimepiride	1mg	4mg, exceptionally 6mg

Table 2.3 Examples of post-prandial regulators

Name	Initial dose	Maximum dose
Repaglinide	0.5–1mg	16mg (4mg tds)
Nateglinide	60mg	180mg tds

Thiazolidinediones also known as glitazones

Introduced as the first oral agent specifically to target insulin resistance.

Mode of action
- Insulin sensitizers that target adipocytes, muscle, and liver cells.
- Enhances insulin sensate genes.
- Increases glucose uptake.
- Increases adipocyte lipogenesis and decrease circulating free fatty acids.

Side effects
- Weight gain.
- Fluid retention.

(See Table 2.4.)

There are also combinations of metformin and the glitazones, these can be particularly useful if the patient is struggling with the number of tablets they need to take and adherence is an issue (see Table 2.5).

Contraindications
Glitazones should be avoided in:
- Cardiac failure or recent history of cardiac failure.
- Renal failure.
- Hepatic impairment, regular liver function test are recommended before commencing treatment and periodically thereafter.
- Severe sepsis.
- Acute alcohol intoxication, alcoholism.
- Pregnancy and breastfeeding.

See BNF for full prescribing information.

Table 2.4 Doses of thiazolidinediones also known as glitazones

Name	Initial dose	Maximum dose
Pioglitazone	15mg	45mg
Rosiglitazone	4mg	8mg

Table 2.5 Combinations of metformin and the glitazones

Name	Initial dose	Maximum dose
Pioglitazone/metformin (Competact®)	15mg/850mg	30mg/1700mg
Rosiglitazone/metformin (Avandamet®)	2mg/500mg	8mg/2g
	4mg/1g	

Alpha-glucosidase inhibitors

Rarely used in the UK due to intolerable side effects. This has limited their use.

Mode of action
- Delay carbohydrate absorption.
- Inhibits breakdown of disaccharidase enzymes, resulting in lower post-prandial glucose levels.

Side effects
- Flatulence.
- Abdominal cramps.
- Diarrhoea.

Initially, small dose are commenced to facilitate tolerance (see Table 2.6).

Contraindications
- Hepatic or severe renal impairment.
- Inflammatory bowel disorders.
- Colonic ulceration.
- Chronic digestive or absorption disorders.

See BNF for full prescribing information.

Table 2.6 Doses of alpha-glucosidase inhibitors

Name	Initial dose	Maximum dose
Acarbose	50mg	600mg

Dipeptidyl peptidase 4 inhibitors (DPP-IV inhibitors)

A new class of oral hypoglycaemic agent.

Mode of action
- Extends the life of GLP1 (incretin mimetic, see 🕮 p. 46).
- Increases insulin production in a glucose dependant manner.
- Reduces hepatic gluoneogenesis.

Side effects
- Gastrointestinal disturbance.
- Increased risk of upper respiratory infection.
- Peripheral oedema.

(See Table 2.7.)

Contraindications
- Ketoacidosis.
- Pregnancy.
- Breast feeding.

See BNF for full prescribing information.

Table 2.7 Examples of DPP-IV inhibitors

Name	Initial dose	Maximum dose
Sitagliptin, for use in combination with metformin or glitazone	100mg	100mg
Vildagliptin	50mg	100mg
Vildagliptin and metformin combination	50mg/850mg	100mg/1700mg

Note that vildagliptin is not licensed for monotherapy.

Oral medications

Oral hypoglycaemic agents have a variety of mechanisms of action to lower blood glucose levels. Each group of oral hypoglycaemic agents target specific organs/tissues to achieve this. See Fig 2.4.

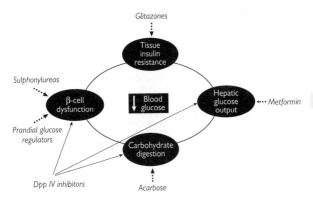

Fig. 2.4 Mechanisms of action of oral hypoglycaemic agents.

Incretin-based therapies

- Incretins are peptide hormones produced in the small intestine.
- GLP1 is secreted in the L cells in the ileum and colon.
- The principle action of GLP1 is to:
  - increase insulin secretion in a glucose dependant manner
  - reduce hepatic gluconeogenesis
  - delay gastric emptying
  - increase satiety.
- In people with Type 2 diabetes, the GLP1 response is significantly reduced or absent.
- The circulating half-life of GLP1 is short due to the rapid degradation by the enzyme dipeptidyl peptidase (DPP-IV).
- Incretin-based therapies seek either to replace deficient levels of GLP1, e.g. exenatide. This is the only incretin-based therapy currently available, although other companies will be launching similar products.

Or

- Prevent the degradation of GLP1 by DPP-IV using DPP-IV inhibitors, e.g. sitagliptin, see Dipeptidyl peptidase 4 inhibitors, p.44.

Action of exenatide

- Enhancing glucose-dependent insulin secretion:
  - exenatide increases, on a glucose dependent basis, the secretion of insulin from pancreatic beta cells
  - as blood glucose concentrations decrease, insulin secretion subsides.
- Suppressing inappropriately elevated glucagon secretion:
  - exenatide suppresses glucagon secretion, which is known to be inappropriately elevated in Type 2 diabetes
  - lower glucagon concentrations lead to decreased hepatic glucose output
  - however, exenatide does not impair the normal glucagon response to hypoglycaemia.
- **Slowing gastric emptying:** exenatide slows gastric emptying thereby reducing the rate at which meal-derived glucose appears in the circulation.
- **Promoting satiety and reducing food intake:** exenatide promotes a feeling of fullness, thereby reducing appetite and food intake.

Clinical questions that inform the decision to commence exenatide

- For use in Type 2 diabetes only for patients on maximum tolerated doses of two or more oral therapies.
- Ideal diabetes duration <15 years (need sustained intrinsic insulin secretion).
- Poor glycaemic control (not associated with weight loss).
- Hba1c >7.5%.
- BMI >35 or gaining weight, despite poor control and lifestyle attempts.
- Not recommended in end-stage renal disease or severe renal impairment.

Initiating exenatide

- The patient should be initiated on 5μg bd for the first month.
- Administer subcutaneously twice daily within 60min before the morning and evening meal (or 2 main meals of the day, approximately 6h or more apart).
- Metformin should be continued.
- If using exenatide in combination with sulphonylureas there is an increased risk of hypoglycaemia, particularly in those patients starting with a lower HbA1c, therefore, consider decreasing sulphonylurea dose by up to 50%.
- It is not licensed for use with glitazones or insulin.
- No increase in blood glucose monitoring is required.
- Review patients on 5μg after 1month and then, if tolerated, the dose should be increased to 10μg bd for the duration of therapy to further improve glycaemic control. If GI side effects are problematic maintain on 5 micrograms bd for another month before attempts at increasing titration.

Side effects

Nausea is the most commonly reported side effect, most episodes being mild to moderate, decreasing over time with most patients.

Explaining exenatide (Byetta) to patients

- All patients will use a Byetta pen device.
- Patients will need to be taught:
  - How to use the pen device
  - Subcutaneous injection technique
  - Storage instructions.

See BNF for full prescribing information, and patient information leaflet supplied with each pen.

Further information

Byetta information packs are available, which contains the following:
- Pocket guide – brief introduction to Byetta.
- Byetta booklet – including 'What is Byetta?' and management of your diabetes.
- Personal diary.
- Quick reference guide – how to use your Byetta pen.

Insulin use in Type 2 diabetes

The majority of patients with Type 2 diabetes will require intensification of treatment, including oral therapies and eventually insulin. The UKPDS demonstrated that 58% of people with Type 2 diabetes required insulin within 14 years of diagnosis (UKPDS 1998). The American Diabetes Association (ADA) and the European Association for the Study of Diabetes (EASD) recommend early initiation of insulin treatment if the individual does not achieve target HbA1c levels (Nathan et al 2006). Insulin initiation in Type 2 diabetes is rarely an immediate requirement unless the individual is acutely unwell; the patient should be an active participant in the decision to commence insulin.

Clinical indications for insulin in Type 2 diabetes

- Inadequate glycaemic control on maximum tolerated oral agents HbA1c above target).
- Symptomatic hyperglycaemia.[1]
- Continual weight loss +/– ketonuria.
- Medical co-morbidities, deteriorating complications of diabetes, cardiovascular disease, deteriorating renal function, etc.
- Recurrent intercurrent illness/infections.
- Pregnancy.

Planning a patient's insulin regimen

There is a wide range of insulin regimens to choose from, but to make an effective decision about which regimen is most appropriate, the following information is required:
- Duration of diabetes.
- Weight and weight change.
- Dietary history.
- Current medical history including treatment.
- Evidence of hyperglycaemic symptoms.
- The patients' personal goals.
- Social and employment history.
- Current glycaemic control based on HbA1c and glucose monitoring profiles.

An assessment of the individuals' physical capabilities, dexterity, eyesight, language and literacy skills are useful in determining the individuals understanding and ability to read supporting materials. The above information will enable the choice of regimen to be tailored to the individual's requirements in terms of preference and lifestyle, as well as achieving clinical outcomes.

There is no evidence-based consensus as to which insulin regimen is the most suitable for Type 2 diabetes and as a result clinical practice varies widely across the UK.

---

1 If the individual is acutely symptomatic, losing weight and presents with ketonuria, insulin needs to be commenced urgently. This may suggest they have Type 1, rather than Type 2 diabetes.

Regimens commonly used in Type 2 diabetes

- Once-daily basal insulin is often given nocte, with a view to fixing the fasting glucose. All oral hypoglycaemic agents are usually continued. with this regimen, although this needs individual assessment.
- Twice daily pre-mixed insulin. Maintain metformin at maximum tolerated dose. Glitazones and sulphonylureas are usually discontinued.

Typically, Type 2 patients are commenced on either of the above regimens, changing to basal bolus if therapeutic goals are not achieved

Starting doses and titration

Insulin is typically initiated at low doses to minimize the risk of hypoglycaemia, this is gradually titrated every 2–3 days based on blood glucose profiles, HbA1c, and agreed targets. See Tables 2.8 and 2.9.

Starting doses: once daily basal insulin – 10units

Table 2.8 Titration guidelines

Fasting blood glucose levels from preceding 2days	Insulin dose change
>10mmol/l	Increase by 8units
>7.8–10mmol/l	Increase by 6units
>6.7–7.8mmol/l	Increase by 4units
>5.6–6.7mmol/l	Increase by 2units
<4.0mmol/l	No change
<3.1mmol/l	Decrease by 2units

Source: Riddle et al (2003).

Starting doses: twice daily premixed – 10units bd

Table 2.9 Titration guidelines, according to blood glucose profiles both doses or one dose may need to be titrated

Blood glucose levels	Insulin dose change
>10mmol/l	Increase by 6units
>7.8–9.9mmol/l	Increase by 4units
>6.1–7.7mmol/l	Increase by 2units
>4.5–6.0mmol/l	No change
<4.5mmol/l	Decrease by 2units

Source: Hirsh et al (2005). See also 📖 p. 62

Determinants of success

- Appropriate regimen chosen to meet therapeutic targets and patient choice/preference.
- Appropriate dose titration.

Risks associated with commencing insulin

- Weight gain.
- **Hypoglycaemia:** clinically actual risk is very low, although a perceived barrier for many patients.
- Non-compliance is a factor that needs to be considered in oral and insulin therapy if targets are to be achieved.

Practicalities of commencing insulin

See 📖 Chapter 5, pp. 81–104.

Specific concerns often raised by people with Type 2 diabetes when commencing insulin

- Social embarrassment/stigma.
- Fear of hypodermic needles.
- Lifestyle changes/restrictions.
- Painful injections.
- Feelings of failure and guilt at not managing their diabetes earlier.
- Becoming more ill as the disease progresses.

Discussing the above topics is essential to allay any concerns, issues, or barriers if insulin therapy is to be successful.

There are many patients who have not achieved glycaemic control on maximum oral medication. Therefore, insulin is a necessary form of treatment in Type 2 diabetes. There is no one regimen that is best for everyone. The choice of regimen should be based on an individualized assessment to ensure success.

Further information

Hirsh IB, Bergenstal EM, Parkin CG, Wright E, Buse JB (2005). A real world approach to insulin therapy in primary care practice. *Clinical Diabetes* **23**(2), 78–86.

Nathan DM, Buse JB, Davidson MB, et al (2006). Management of hyperglycaemia in Type 2 diabetes: A consensus algorithm for the initiation and adjustment of therapy. A consensus statement from the ADA & EASD. *Diabetes Care* **29**(8), 1963–72.

Riddle MC, Rosenstock J, Gerich J (2003). The treat-to-target trial: randomized addition of glargine or human NPH insulin to oral therapy of type 2 diabetic patients. *Diabetes Care* **26**(3), 3080-3086.

United Kingdom Prospective Diabetes Study (1998). Intensive blood-glucose control with sulpho-nylurea or insulin compared with conventional treatment and risk of complications in patients with type 2 diabetes (UKPDS 33). *Lancet* **352**(9131), 837–53.

Addressing adherence

Type 2 diabetes is a progressive condition that requires intensification of treatment. To achieve blood glucose, bp, and lipid targets, increasing numbers of medications are needed. Non-adherence to dietary and lifestyle changes have been well documented, and non-adherence to diabetes medication is potentially one of the most serious problems facing diabetes care delivery.

Studies have suggested that adherence is a bigger problem with the elderly and when therapy is prescribed long-term, as it is with diabetes. Alongside this, there appears to be a relationship between the frequency of doses taken and adherence. Once daily medications may be beneficial in these circumstances

Compliance aids supplied by pharmacies can also be a useful tool to aid adherence.

Poor adherence may result from:
- Poor understanding of the importance of managing diabetes.
- Poor understanding of medications and their actions.
- Experience of side effects.
- Health beliefs relating to taking medications.
- Lack of perceived benefit particularly if patients feel well.

It is essential when reviewing patients to ascertain adherence to medications, and there is no effective intervention to assess adherence other than discussing with patients in a non-judgemental way, ensuring patients are fully aware of the action of their medications and when to take them. Assess for any side effects of medications that may prevent patients from taking them. The majority of general practice computer systems can indicate if a patient is not collecting sufficient prescriptions to fulfil their prescribed doses.

Poor adherence is a major obstacle to the benefit of complex therapy regimens used in the treatment of Type 2 diabetes, patients need to be fully aware of this and engaged in any decision-making regarding the addition of any new medications.

Type 1 diabetes

Incidence and epidemiology

Type 1 diabetes accounts for approximately 10–15% of diagnosed diabetes. The frequency of Type 1 diabetes is increasing. In Europe the estimated increase is 3–4% with the highest increase being seen in children diagnosed under the age of 5 years (Pickup & Williams 2004).

There are wide variations in the incidence of Type 1 diabetes between populations with high frequencies, such as in Finland and Sweden, and low frequencies, such as some areas in China.

It has been suggested that the variability in incidence is linked to:
• Environmental factors.
• Genetic factors.

Further information

Pickup J, Williams G (2004). *Handbook of diabetes*. Blackwell Publishing: Oxford.

Aetiology

Type 1 diabetes is caused by absolute insulin deficiency. The aetiology of Type 1 diabetes is complex and not fully understood, although it is identified that an autoimmune destruction of the Islet of Langerhans beta cells occurs (Fig. 3.1). It is thought that environmental influences may trigger this destruction in those with a genetic predisposition to Type 1 diabetes. Although of those developing Type 1 diabetes only 10–15% will have a family history, the majority of cases occurring are completely sporadic.

Insulitis and auto-antibodies

The autoimmune destruction of the beta cells is seen in chronic inflammation of the beta cells, known as insulitis. The degree of insulitis can be measured by Islet cell auto-antibodies (ICA) and glutamic acid decarboxylase (GAD) antibodies.

Not everybody with Islet cell antibodies develops Type 1 diabetes, suggesting that insulitis does not necessarily lead to sufficient beta cells becoming damaged and Type 1 diabetes developing. However, the risk is much higher if both ICA and GAD are present.

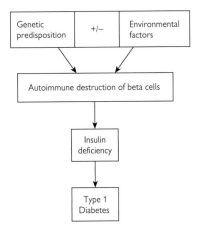

Fig. 3.1 Aetiology of Type 1 diabetes.

Presentation

Type 1 diabetes tends to occur in the younger age group with the majority of patients developing it under the age of 40 years. The onset is typically acute with symptoms of hyperglycaemia evident at diagnosis.

Clinical features of Type 1 diabetes
- Usually diagnosed <40 years of age.
- Symptoms of hyperglycaemia evident.
- Normal weight, but often with evidence of recent weight loss.
- Absolute insulin deficiency.
- Ketones often present in the urine.

Late onset Type 1 diabetes
This is also referred to as latent autoimmune diabetes of adults (LADA). Increasingly, late onset Type 1 diabetes is being recognized. Clinical features are:
- Onset >40 years of age.
- May be moderately overweight, e.g. BMI around 27.
- Poor response to sulphonylurea therapy.
- Co-existent autoimmune diseases typically thyroid disorders.
- Definitive diagnosis can be made by the presence of anti-GAD antibodies.

It is essential to establish a correct diagnosis. The differences in the characteristics of Type 1 and Type 2 diabetes are detailed in Table 3.1.

Table 3.1 Characteristics of Type 1 and Type 2 diabetes mellitus

Characteristic	Type 1	Type 2
Insulin status	Insulin secretion depleted	Deviations in insulin secretion
Age	Under 40s usually	40+ or any age
Presentation	Rapid onset	Slow onset
Body	Underweight or normal	80–90% diagnosed cases overweight
Family history	Weak	Strong
Islet cell antibodies	Present	Absent
Symptoms	Polyuria, polydipsia, weight loss	Asymptomatic or as Type 1
Ketones/ketosis	Present or prone	Rare
Frequency	15% of diagnosed cases	85% of diagnosed cases
Complications	Common related to duration and contributing risk factors	Sometimes present at diagnosis. Common related to duration and contributing risk factors
Treatment	Insulin, diet, exercise	Diet, oral agents, insulin, exercise

Aims of treatment

Initial aim
The initial aim of treatment is to save life:
- Insulin is essential for life, without it ketoacidosis, coma, and death will occur (see 📖 Diabetic ketoacidosis, p. 172).
- Relief of symptoms and reverse ketosis.

Intermediate and long-term aims of treatment
- To maintain quality of life.
- To achieve blood glucose levels, bp, and lipid profiles to target levels according to national and international guidelines.
- Reduce risk of micro- and macrovascular complications.
- Keep risk of hypoglycaemia at minimum.

Types of insulin

Insulin preparations can be divided into 3 main groups:
- Short/rapid-acting insulin (see Tables 3.2 and 3.3).
- Intermediate and long-acting insulin (see Tables 3.3 and 3.4).
- Long-acting analog insulins (see Table 3.5).
- Pre-mixed insulin (see Tables 3.6 and 3.7).

Most insulins are now human synthetic formulations. Although some preparations of animal insulin are available, the use of these is in decline in the UK. It would be rare to commence a newly diagnosed patient on an animal insulin.

Table 3.2 Types of insulin: rapid-acting analog insulins

Name	Duration of action
Insulin aspart: Novorapid® Insulin lispro: Humalog® Insulin glulisine: Apidra®	Injected immediately before meals or with meals, onset of action within 10–15min, peak action 2h and duration up to 3–5h

Table 3.3 Types of insulin: short-acting insulins

Name	Duration of action
Humulin S® Actrapid® Insuman® rapid	Injected 15–30min before meals, onset of action 30–60min, peak action 2–6h and duration up to 12h.

Table 3.4 Types of insulin: intermediate and long-acting insulins

Name	Duration of action
Insulatard® Humulin I® Insuman Basal®	When injected depending on the insulin chosen onset of action is approximately 1–2h, maximal effect 2–8h and duration 18–24h. Typically given before breakfast and or bedtime

Table 3.5 Types of insulin: long-acting analog insulins

Name	Duration of action
Insulin glargine: Lantus®	When injected depending on the insulin chosen onset of action is approximately 1–2h, maximal effect 22–24h
Insulin detemir: Levemir®	Typically given before bed, but can be given before breakfast

Table 3.6 Types of insulin: biphasic insulins pre-mixed combinations of short- and intermediate-acting insulins

Name	Duration of action
Humulin M3® Mixtard 30® Insuman Comb 15® Insuman Comb 30® Insuman Comb 50®	When injected depending on the insulin chosen onset of action is approximately 30min, maximal effect 4–12h, and a duration 12–18h. Typically given pre breakfast and evening meal

Table 3.7 Types of insulin: biphasic analog insulins pre-mixed combinations of rapid-acting analog and intermediate-acting insulins

Name	Duration of action
Humalog Mix25® Humalog Mix50® Novomix 30®	When injected, depending on the insulin chosen, onset of action is within 15min and duration of action is up to 24h.

Onset of action, peak effect, and duration are only approximate as individual patient variations will occur.

See current BNF for full prescribing information.

Insulin absorption

Subcutaneous insulins are injected as hexamers, which is the stable form of the insulin molecule. The hexamer is too large to be absorbed into the blood stream, In order to be absorbed into the blood stream; the hexamers need to diffuse and dilute in order to become much smaller (monomers). In traditional insulins the process is slower as the hexamers initially become dimers before monomers. The rapid-acting analogue insulins move to monomers straight after the hexamer stage, enabling more rapid absorption (see Fig. 3.2).

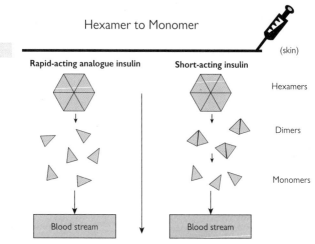

Fig. 3.2 Insulin absorption.

Treatment of Type 1 diabetes

Treatment for Type 1 diabetes includes:
- Physiological insulin replacement.
- Self-blood glucose monitoring.
- Diet and lifestyle modifications.
- Structured education.

Physiological insulin replacement

The aim of insulin replacement therapy in a patient with Type 1 diabetes is to mimic as closely as possible normal endogenous insulin production. This consists of a constant delivery of insulin to manage hepatic glucose output and a peak of insulin after meals to limit post-prandial hyperglycaemia. This can be achieved by 4 injections a day, consisting of a background insulin, often referred to as basal insulin given nocte (at night) and 3 injections with meals referred to as bolus insulin. In the DCCT (1993), a basal bolus regimen or insulin pump therapy was compared with a bd mixed insulin, alongside intensive education. The basal/bolus or pump insulin led to the achievement of an Hba1c at 7.2%. This was linked to a significant reduction in the long-term complications associated with diabetes (see 📖 Chapter 9, pp. 179–218).

At diagnosis, some patients may not wish to commence 4 injections per day. In this instance, twice daily pre-mixed insulins may be used.

Initially, small doses are commenced to reduce the risk of hypoglycaemia. In some areas, specialist teams commence ½–1unit of insulin per kg of the patients weight.

Advantages of a basal bolus regimen

- Mimics as closely as possible, via injections, endogenous insulin production.
- Flexibility of meal sizes and times.

Disadvantages of a basal bolus regimen

- 4–5 injections per day.
- Frequent blood glucose monitoring to enable suitable adjustment of insulin doses according to meals and activity, etc.

Practicalities of giving insulin

See 📖 Chapter 5, pp. 81–104.

Dietary aspects of Type 1 diabetes

Alongside the current dietary recommendations for diabetes, Type 1 patients are increasingly being taught to count carbohydrate intake and adjust their insulin accordingly. This is known as the insulin to carbohydrate ratio. This is reached by a simple calculation. Typically, 1unit of insulin per 10g of carbohydrate is given. This allows more flexibility in terms of the type and quantity of carbohydrate eaten.

Weight loss is often a presenting feature of Type 1 diabetes. When insulin is commenced, many patients complain of an increased appetite. This is normal and patients are encouraged to eat according to appetite, and

their weight often returns to their pre-diagnosis weight as the body is able to store fat and utilize glucose for energy.

Self-blood glucose monitoring in Type 1 diabetes

People with Type 1 diabetes are subject to a wider variability of blood glucose levels and are at an increased risk of hypoglycaemia. Therefore, frequent blood glucose monitoring is recommended. Frequent monitoring of blood glucose levels enables the person with Type 1 diabetes to:

- Adjust insulin doses according to carbohydrate intake, therefore allowing more flexibility with meals.
- Prepare for and manage blood glucose levels when preparing for activity.
- Adjust insulin doses according to trends and patterns of blood glucose monitoring.
- Optimize blood glucose levels to achieve target pre- and post-prandial blood glucose levels and target HbA1c result.
- Reduce risk of hypoglycaemia.

See 📖 Chapter 7, pp. 119–160, for more information on blood glucose monitoring.

Structured education and Type 1 diabetes

Type 1 is a complex condition for the individual to manage, a range of self-management skills are necessary to achieve a balance between optimal diabetes control and minimizing the impact on daily life as much as possible. Structured education programmes are being developed across the country to achieve this. See 📖 Structured education: meeting NICE criteria, p. 106.

Topics typically included in these programmes

- Developing an understanding of Type 1 diabetes.
- Practical skills, such as self-injection and blood glucose monitoring.
- Diet including carbohydrate counting.
- Lifestyle issues.
- Self-adjustment of insulin.
- Management of hypo- and hyperglycaemia.
- Management of Type 1 diabetes during illness/stress.

Further information

Dose Adjustment For Normal Eating (DAFNE). 🖳 http://www.dafne.uk.com

Shearer A, Bagust A, Sanderson D et al. (2004) Cost effectiveness of flexible intensive insulin management to enable dietary freedom in people with Type 1 diabetes. *Diabetic Med* **21**, 460–7.

Alternative methods of insulin delivery

Inhaled insulin

The lungs provide a highly vascular absorptive surface, making them suitable for the use of insulin, which has been manufactured in a dry powder formulation. Efficacy is comparable with subcutaneous injection and tolerability is good. At present, inhaled insulin is not available in the UK, although there are some products in development.

Continuous subcutaneous infusion of insulin (CSII)

- A portable pump is used to deliver subcutaneous insulin at variable rates, which mimics endogenous insulin production more closely than any other method of delivering insulin.
- A basal rate of insulin is delivered throughout the 24h and this can be altered to match the patients' insulin requirements. The patient activates the pump to deliver bolus doses of insulin at meal times according to carbohydrate intake.
- CSII can achieve excellent metabolic control.

See 📖 Insulin pumps: continuous subcutaneous insulin infusion, p. 88, for futher details.

Chapter 4

Dietary treatment for diabetes

Diet and diabetes

Diet is an integral part of diabetes management and should be tailored to each individual. The aims of dietary advice are to:
- Reduce primary symptoms of diabetes.
- To help optimize glycaemic control.
- To help ↓ the risk of complications through lipid and bp management.
- Ensure a nutritionally adequate diet.
- Management of weight.
- Quality of life.

Steps to dietary management

- Keep as active as possible.
- Regular meals to include a moderate portion of starchy carbohydrate (CHO) at each meal.
- Maintaining a varied diet including food choices from all food groups – CHOs, protein, and fat.
- Aiming for 5 portions of fruit and vegetables a day.
- ↓ Intake of sucrose and refined CHO foods in line with general healthy eating.
- Encouraging more low glycaemic index (GI) food choices (see ▢ Glycaemic Index, p. 76).
- ↓ Total fat intake – reduction especially of saturated fat, whilst encouraging mono-unsaturated fats.
- ↓ Salt intake.
- Alcohol in moderation.
- Aiming for a healthy weight or maintaining weight.
- Avoid 'diabetic' products.

Carbohydrates

Less sucrose and sucrose-containing foods, such as cakes, biscuits, confectionery, sweet drinks, etc., will help optimize glycaemic and lipid (tryglyceride) control (see ▢ Carbohydrates, p. 74).

Encourage low glycaemic index food (see ▢ Glycaemic Index, p. 76).

Fat

Replace saturated fats (found in animal fat and dairy products) with mono-unsaturated fat (found in olive and rapeseed oil) where possible. Encourage a decrease of pies and pastries, biscuits and cakes to optimize glycaemia, lipid (cholesterol), and weight management.

Encourage oily fish once or twice a week, or 2–3 times a week if patient has had myocardial infarction (MI).

Protein

Protein intake may need to be monitored in some cases of nephropathy, but specialist dietetic advice should be taken.

Fruit and vegetables

Aiming for at least five portions of fruit and vegetables daily will ensure an optimum intake of vitamins, minerals, and antioxidants. A portion would be:

- 3 tablespoons vegetables or tinned or stewed fruit.
- A small bowl of salad.
- A piece of fresh fruit (one apple, one pear, handful grapes or berries, small banana).
- 150ml fruit juice (only one glass a day can count as a portion of fruit).

Salt

Limit salt to 5g/day for women and 7g/day for men (approximately 1 level teaspoon) a day. Avoid salt substitutes.

Activity

Encourage regular activity. Where appropriate, recommend 30min a day, which can be taken in short time blocks, gradually getting longer.

Further information

Diabetes UK ◫ www.diabetes.org.uk.

The British Diabetic Association ◫ www.bda.uk.com.

Food Standards Agency-Food Labelling ◫ www.food.gov.uk/foodlabelling.

Nutritional Subcommittee of the Diabetes Care Advisory Committee of Diabetes UK (2003). The implementation of nutritional advice for people with diabetes. *Diabetic Med* **20**, 786–807.

Weight management

Weight management is fundamental to good glycaemic control, especially for T2 diabetes. Obesity and particularly central obesity is a risk factor for developing insulin resistance and T2 diabetes. Being overweight is classed as having a body mass index (BMI) >25kg/m² or waist circumference of >94cm (male), >80cm female. See Table 4.1.

Table 4.1 Waist circumference risk

Sex	Increased risk	High risk
Male	94cm (37ins)	102cm (40ins)
Female	80cm (32ins)	88cm (35ins)

Medications that may cause weight gain
- Antipsychotics and antidepressants.
- Corticosteroids.
- Beta blockers.
- Oral hypoglycaemic agents (sulphonylureas, meglitinides and glitazones).
- Insulin.
- Anticonvulsants.

Weight loss
5–10% weight loss in conjunction with regular activity of at least 30min/day can reduce insulin resistance and improve blood glucose and lipid profiles.

A 100kcal reduction a day can help to ↓ weight by 4–5kg (8–11lb) in a year (1 digestive biscuit contains 70kcal).

Lifestyle advice
- **Motivation**: overweight people need to be motivated to achieve effective weight loss.
- **Aim for small changes** at a time and gradually build on these once confidence and motivation are achieved.
- **Think positive**: concentrate on what can be eaten more of, rather than what should be eaten less of.
- **Encourage regular activity**: at least 30min a day where appropriate.
- **Encourage regular meals** (skipping meals can lead to weight gain).
- **Encourage healthy eating.**
- **Encourage slow weight loss** (up to 1kg /1–2lb a week) as it is more likely weight will stay off.
- **Preventing further weight gain** is a preferable outcome to continuing to gain weight.
- Refer to specialist registered dietician for **portion control advice**.

Carbohydrate counting

Some people with diabetes may be on basal bolus (four injections a day) or on insulin pumps (continuous subcut infusion of insulin).

Basal bolus (see Table 4.2)

- **Basal insulin** (Lantus®, Levemir®, Insulatard®): long-acting insulin injected either before bed or at breakfast – sometimes a split dose at breakfast and bed-time.
- **Bolus insulin** (Novorapid®, Humalog®, Humulin S®): quick-acting insulin injected at each meal of the day.

Insulin pump

- Pre set continuous delivery of basal (quick-acting) insulin.
- Boluses of quick-acting insulin delivered when eating.

The mealtime insulin for the above two methods of diabetes management is adjusted according to the CHO content of the meals and activity levels – CHO counting.

Table 4.2 Basal bolus

Benefits	Considerations
Flexible meal patterns	Four or more injections a day with basal bolus
Can choose what and when to eat – gives more freedom with food	Possibly injecting in front of others
Eating out is less problematic	More frequent blood glucose monitoring
More flexibility with timing of insulin – can be given after eating a meal	Calculating CHO content of food
Can delay or skip meals (but not encouraged as part of healthy eating message)	Calculating insulin doses to give with food
No need to snack	Understanding how to adjust insulin for activity and food
Can help manage activity	Takes time
High blood glucose levels may be corrected at meal times	Basal insulin needs to be right before blousing works effectively

Seek professional specialist diabetes dietetic advice for CHO counting advice for people on basal bolus or on insulin pumps. T1 group education courses such as DAFNE (Dose Adjustment For Normal Eating) are available, but seek advice from local diabetes centre for further information of courses available locally.

Glycaemic Index

The glycaemic index (GI) is a ranking of the speed of onset of CHO foods (see 📖 Carbohydrates, p. 74) and their effect on blood glucose levels (Table 4.3).

- Carbohydrates that are broken down quickly have a **high GI**. These foods cause a rapid rise in blood glucose levels.
- Carbohydrates that are broken down slowly have a **low GI**. These foods cause a more gradual and controlled rise in blood glucose levels.

What are the benefits of the GI?

- Meals based on low GI help manage blood glucose levels. This will help with diabetes control.
- Low GI foods help satiety and so can aid appetite. This helps less to be eaten and so can help with weight management.
- Low GI diets may help reduce the risk of heart disease and improve cholesterol levels.
- Can be useful for people participating in sporting activities.

Considerations

- The GI does not take into consideration quantity. Large portions of low GI foods can result in high blood glucose levels.
- High fat foods have a low GI as fat slows down gastric emptying and the rate of digestion, and so delays the rate at which CHO is digested and absorbed into the blood stream. Too much fat will contribute to weight gain (which may have an effect on diabetes management) and will also have an effect on lipids. High fat foods should therefore be limited.
- Large quantities of protein may also slow down gastric emptying, and so slow down the rate at which CHO is digested and absorbed into the blood stream. Protein is to be encouraged in moderation.

Key points

- Eat regular meals.
- Include low GI foods at each meal, especially if including high GI foods.
- Encourage similar quantities of CHOs at each meal.
- High fat high protein meals can result in weight gain and high blood glucose levels.
- Including a low GI food after a meal as a dessert can help with blood glucose and weight management.
- Seek professional dietetic advice for guidance on how to use the GI effectively.

Table 4.3 Glycaemic index values of different food types

	Low GI	Medium GI	High GI
Breads	Multigrain, rye bread	Pitta bread, (white, wholemeal), wholemeal bread, muffins, crumpets, malt loaf	White bread, baguette
Biscuits	Oatmeal biscuits	Rich tea, digestives, shortbread	Crackers, morning coffee, vanilla wafer
Cereals	Porridge, Special K, Allbran	Shredded Wheat	Sultana Bran, Rice Krispies, Cornflakes, sugary cereals, e.g. Coco Pops
Grains and pasta	Pasta, buckwheat, bulgar wheat, oatmeal biscuits	Basmati rice, couscous, quinoa	Brown and white rice, rice cakes, crackers
Potato	Sweet potato	Boiled potatoes, new potatoes	French fries, instant potato, roasted potato, mashed potato
Vegetables and pulses	Peas, lentils, beans (e.g. baked, kidney), carrots, yam, tomato juice	Beetroot	Parsnips, broad beans, popcorn
Fruit	Apples, pears, citrus, kiwi, cherries, plums, grapes, dried pear, dried apricots, dried peaches, mango, prunes	Mixed dried fruit, fresh apricot, fruit juice, sultanas, banana, raisins, dried figs	Dried dates, melons, jam and marmalade
Dairy	Low fat milk, diet yoghurt, ice-cream, low-fat custard, Yakult light, Vitasoy soya milk		Vitasoy calcium enriched rice milk
Miscellaneous	Dark chocolate, peanuts, cashew nuts, tomato juice, marmalade – no added sugar	Honey, reduced sugar jams	Sugar, glucose tablets, soft drinks, sweets, e.g. jelly beans, marmalade

Understanding food labels

Food labels can be very confusing. When reading food labels think about how often and how much of the food is eaten, and how it fits into the overall diet. Food labels provide a lot of information, but the relatively new traffic light system has made understanding this information less complicated.

- Green = low
- Amber = medium
- Red = high

The traffic light system informs at a glance if the food is high, medium, or low in fat, saturated fat, salt, and sugar, and so can help to make healthier food choices (see Fig. 4.1).
- The more green lights there are the healthier the food choice.
- Products with amber labels mean the food choice is fine to have, but try to include plenty of the green as well.
- Red means the food choice is high in a nutrient or nutrients that should generally, for healthy eating, be eaten in smaller quantities.
- For healthy food choices, encourage more products with green and amber labels, and fewer products with red labels.

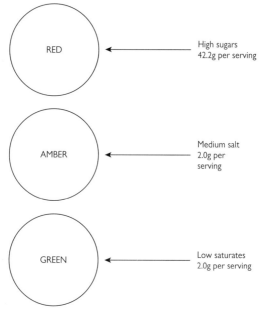

Fig. 4.1 Traffic light system.

The nutrition label

Most food packages will provide a nutritional breakdown of the product. This can help with making healthy food choices. The label will always give the nutrition information 'per 100g' and usually per portion. When looking at snacks, compare the 'per 100g' and the 'per portion' for complete meals (see Table 4.4).

Table 4.4 Nutritional label values per 100g

A LOT (these amounts or more)	A LITTLE (these amounts or less)
10g sugars	2g sugars
20g fat	3g fat
5g saturates	1g saturates
0.5g sodium	0.1g sodium

To calculate the salt content of a product:
g Sodium × 2.5 = g salt (1g sodium = 2.5g salt)
Daily guideline for salt is 7g for men and 5g for women.

Nutrition information explained

Energy

This is measured either in kJ and/or kcal (calories). Recommended daily amounts are approximately 2500kcal for men and 2000kcal for women.

Carbohydrate/starch/sugar

The total CHO includes both starch and sugar. Most of the energy in the diet should come from starch. 'Of which sugars' refers to the amount of CHO that is sugar, both natural and added.

Reduced sugar contains 25% less sugar than an equivalent standard variety. *Low sugar* contains no more than 5g sugars per 100g or per serving if a normal serving is >100g). *No added sugar/unsweetened* only contains sugar that occurs naturally in the food. Sugar-free contains no more than 0.2g sugars per 100g/100ml.

Fat

Can be split into 3 types of fat – saturated, mono-unsaturated, and poly-unsaturated. Too much saturated fat may increase cholesterol levels. Encourage less total saturated fat and choose mono-unsaturated or poly-unsaturated fat if possible. Remember that all fat carries calories and too much of any type of fat may lead to weight gain. *Reduced fat* contains 25% less fat than an original product. *Low fat* contains no more than 3g fat per 100g. *Fat free* contains no more than 0.15g fat per 100g.

Recommended daily amounts for men are approximately 95g, and 70g for women.

Fibre

Daily guideline for healthy eating:
• **Men:** 20g/day.
• **Women:** 16g/day.

Chapter 5

Practical skills

Practical skills overview

Diabetes is a chronic condition and it is important that the person with diabetes becomes an expert in their own care. There are a range of practical skills that are necessary for the patient with diabetes to master. Depending on the Type of diabetes, the skills may vary.

It is important these skills are reviewed to ensure best practice is maintained. An ideal time to carry out this review is during the annual review process (see Annual review: interpreting results and target ranges, p. 120).

Self-management skills: insulin

Practicalities of giving insulin

Insulin is inactivated by gastrointestinal (GI) enzymes and must therefore be given by injection into the subcutaneous tissue, from where it is absorbed.

The needle lengths have been developed to ensure subcutaneous injection when injected at an angle of 90° to the skin surface. It may be necessary to pinch up the skin in the lean patient to avoid intramuscular injection and ensure an injection into subcutaneous tissue (see Fig. 5.1).

Insulin needles have been designed for single use only. Some patients choose to re-use the needles. Whilst this is unlikely to cause infections at sites, it is thought to increase subcutaneous trauma as the needle loses its sharpness. This may contribute to the development of complications at injection sites, as scar tissue may form, making injections increasingly difficult over time.

Injection sites

Insulin may be given into the abdomen, thigh, or buttocks. Typically, patients use the abdomen or thighs as self-injecting into the buttocks does require a certain amount of dexterity and suppleness. Absorption of insulin varies marginally from each site, so it is suggested that injection sites be rotated to allow adjustments for this variation. It is not necessary to clean the skin with alcohol or antiseptic as insulin has an antibacterial property and infections at injection sites are rare. Maintaining some consistency when injecting into sites is recommended.

Factors that influence insulin absorption

- Exercising an area after injection.
- Massaging the area round the injection site.
- Angle and depth of injection, such as injecting into muscle.
- Insulin not resuspended correctly.
- Complications at injection sites such as lipohypertrophy.
- Temperature of injection site.
- Smoking.

Site rotation

To prevent any complications at injection sites, site rotation is important. Site rotation means rotating within the site. For example, if a patient always gives their breakfast insulin into the thighs, they should use alternate thighs and choose a different place to inject at that site. Advising the patient to inject within the same anatomical region may reduce daily variations in absorption and metabolic control. This not only contributes to the consistency of insulin absorption, but also reduces the risk of complications at injections sites, such as lipohypertrophy (see 📖 Glossary, pp. 357–360).

Storage

Insulin is best given at room temperature and insulin in use can be stored for up to 4 weeks at room temperature (at not more than 25°C). If the ambient temperature is warmer than this, a cool bag should be used Insulins not in use should be kept in the refrigerator and expiry dates should be checked prior to use.

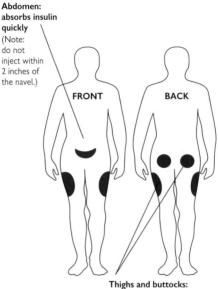

Fig. 5.1 Insulin injection sites. Adapted from Matthews D et al (2008), *Diabetes*, with permission from Oxford University Press.

Devices, needles, and sharps disposal

Injection devices known as 'pen devices' are the most common way for people to self-inject insulin. These can be durable and filled with insulin cartridges, and some insulins are available in disposable pen devices. Regardless of whether a preloaded or durable device is used, the individuals should be informed of the following:

- The expiry date of the insulin should be checked.
- There should be sufficient insulin in the cartridge and it should be the right insulin for the right injection time. Insulins can look very similar – the majority of long-acting analogue insulins are now clear; therefore, as all rapid/short-acting insulins are also clear it would be easy to mistake the insulins and use the incorrect insulin type.
- If a cloudy insulin is used, it needs to be re-suspended before injection. It should be rolled in the palms of the hands and inverted upside down 2–3 times. This ensures that the glass bead inside the cartridge moves to help ensure thorough resuspension and should be done until the mixture is uniformly cloudy or milky in appearance.
- A new needle should be used every time. Pen needles and disposable syringes are designed for single use – repeated use can lead to pain and discomfort during the injection.
- How the pen works, in terms of loading, dialling, and resetting the dose if the incorrect dose is dialled, and finally how to deliver a dose.
- As preparation for the actual dose of insulin, a test shot/dose of approximately 2units should be expelled from the insulin pen to ensure it is correctly primed and the needle is not blocked.
- Safe disposal of sharps is of paramount importance. Local guidelines may differ. Please check with the local council.
- A needle clipping device is available on prescription (see Fig. 5.2).
- For those patients who find it difficult to self-inject there are some automatic pen devices available such as PenMate® (Novo Nordisk Ltd), which attaches to a NovoPen® 3 and demi, and provides automatic injection of insulin. MHI 500 is a needle-less injector.
- True needle phobia is extremely rare. The majority of patients self-inject without any problem.

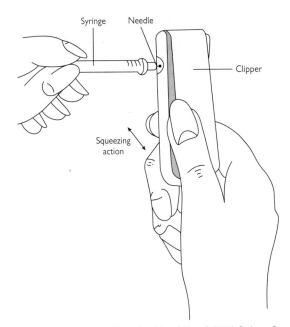

Syringe Needle

Clipper

Squeezing
action

Fig. 5.2 Needle clippers in use. Reproduced from Hillson R (2008), *Diabetes Care*, with permission from Rowan Hillson.

Further information

Hillson R (2008). *Diabetes Care: A Practical Manual*. Oxford University Press, Oxford.

Insulin pumps: continuous subcutaneous insulin infusion

A portable pump is used to deliver subcutaneous insulin at variable rates, mimicking endogenous insulin production more closely than any other method of delivering insulin.

A basal rate of insulin is delivered throughout the 24h and this can be altered to match the patient's insulin requirements. The patient activates the pump to deliver bolus doses of insulin at meal times according to CHO intake.

CSII can achieve excellent metabolic control.

The expense of insulin pumps limits their widespread use in the UK. NICE recommend this as a treatment option for adults and children over 12 years old with Type 1 diabetes, and these individuals need to meet the following criteria (NICE 2008):
- Attempts to achieve target HbA1c, on basal bolus regimes experience disabling hypoglycaemia, defined as repeated and unpredictable hypos that result in persistent anxiety about re-occurrence and significantly affects quality of life.

Or
- HbA1c levels remain >8.5% on basal bolus therapy (multiple daily injections – MDI), including if appropriate the use of long-acting analogue insulins.
- Basal bolus therapy (MDI) is considered impractical or inappropriate.
- It is not recommended for Type 2 diabetes.

Benefits of pump therapy
- More physiological replacement of insulin.
- Fewer glycaemic excursions.
- Reduction of HbA1c.
- Reduced hypoglycaemia.
- Improvement in hypoglycaemia unawareness.
- Reduced insulin dose.
- Insulin adjustment more accurate.
- Fewer injections.
- Increased flexibility and the ability to be more spontaneous in daily life.
- Improved quality of life.

Limitations of pump therapy

- Each pump costs between £2000 and £3000, and consumables cost approximately £1000 per annum. This is £1000 above the cost of standard insulin therapy.
- The pump is attached to the individual all of the time.
- Reliance on technology.
- Intensive blood glucose (BG) monitoring is required.
- Potential for skin infections at cannula site.
- Giving sets are prone to blockage.
- Requires significant time and effort to manage diabetes on pump therapy.

Further information

NICE (2008). *NICE technology appraisal 57*. NICE, London.

Commencing pump therapy

Insulin pumps are connected to a giving set and a cannula, which is sited subcutaneously on the abdominal wall. The cannula and giving set must be changed at least every 3 days, or before this if BG control deteriorates because of problems with the injection site, giving set, or cannula, if redness occurs around the site, if the giving set or cannula become dislodged, or if blood is seen tracking back into the set.

Starting doses of insulin

Basal rates

The mean total daily doses of insulin previously taken. This is reduced by 30% before calculating the doses of insulin on pump therapy, e.g.

- Breakfast soluble   8 units
- Lunch soluble   10 units
- Evening meal soluble   16 units
- Nocte basal insulin   26 units
- Total dose taken prior to using pump   60 units
- Total daily pump dose   60 units (30%)
- The new total insulin dose   42 units*

*50% of this is given as the basal insulin.

The 21 units is divided by 24hr = 0.8 units per hr.

General principles: for the first 24h only one basal rate is started as per above, which can be adjusted based on BG results, the majority of pumps enable variable basal rates based on the individuals needs.

Bolus doses

The dose of insulin required for CHO intake is based on the 500 rule; the total daily pump dose of insulin is divided by 500, e.g. total daily pump dose in the above example is 500/42 units = 11.9.

Carbohydrate bolus = 1 unit of insulin for every 12g CHO. In this example the majority of healthcare professionals would suggest using 1 unit per 10g CHO for ease of calculation.

Correction doses

Correction doses are given if BG level targets are outside of the range expected for the individual. They may be given either before a meal to correct high BG or after meals.

The correction dose is calculated based on the 100 rule. Divide total daily pump dose into 100, e.g. 100/42 units = 2.3. This figure is the amount by which 1 unit of insulin will reduce BG and, for ease of application, are usually rounded up to the nearest whole unit, in this example, 1 unit of insulin will reduce the BG level by 2mmol.

The above dose calculations may be subject to change depending on the locality and it is worth checking local protocols/guidelines.

Using pump therapy enables the individual with BG monitoring skills to adjust their insulin doses more accurately, responding to and anticipating CHO intake, prevailing BG levels, and activity. However, this does require the individual to be motivated and committed to managing their diabetes in this way. Insulin pump therapy is not an easy option. Improvements in quality of life have been demonstrated, by increasing flexibility autonomy and socialization. Alongside this the reduction in disabling hypoglycaemia is of significant benefit.

Disconnecting insulin pumps

Insulin pumps use only rapid-acting insulin so when disconnected the BG levels will rise as soon as the last dose of insulin is absorbed. Disconnection is only recommended for periods of ½h or less to prevent a rapid increase in BG levels. Often this time is sufficient for a shower/ bath or short activity. All of the pumps are robust enough for their continued use during sport and some pumps are even waterproof.

Pump alarms

All of the current insulin pumps are sophisticated and incorporate an audible alarm if insulin delivery is interrupted. This includes:

- Occlusion of cannula.
- Batteries running low.
- Insulin reservoir low.
- Mechanical failure.

Individuals must be taught not to rely solely on alarms for indications of pump failure, as the most effective way of assessing if an insulin pump is working is by regular BG monitoring. This will alert the user if there is a potential problem with the pump or delivery of insulin. If the cannula becomes displaced from the site of injection, the pump alarm will not necessarily sound. The user may also not notice immediately as such small quantities of insulin are being delivered; it will only be when BG levels are taken that a problem may become apparent.

NICE recommends that insulin pump therapy is only initiated by trained specialist teams, which include a physician with a special interest in pump therapy, a diabetes nurse specialist, and a dietician. They should provide structured education programmes, and advice on diet, lifestyle, and exercise for individuals using pump therapy.

Further information

Insulin Pumpers UK ☐ www.insulin-pumpers.org.uk
NICE (2008). *NICE technology appraisal 57*. NICE, London.

Blood glucose monitoring: overview

Blood glucose monitoring

Research has shown that self-monitoring BG is an important tool both for improving glycaemic control and in empowering people with Type 1 and Type 2 diabetes to be expert in managing their own condition.

NICE 2008 recommend self-monitoring BG should be available to:
- Individuals treated with insulin.
- Individuals on oral hypoglycaemic agents to provide information on hypoglycaemia.
- Assess changes in glucose control resulting from medications and lifestyle changes.
- Monitor changes during inter-current illness.
- To ensure safety during activities, including driving.
- For individuals with newly diagnosed Type 2 diabetes, self-monitoring BG should be offered only as an integral part of self-management education.

Irrespective of how long a person has been self-monitoring or how well they were taught, it is essential to check their BG monitoring technique to ensure they are:
- Obtaining a sample of capillary blood.
- Correctly using the BG meter.
- Recording and interpreting results correctly.
- Cleaning and checking the accuracy of the BG meter.

Blood glucose monitoring technique: obtaining a sample of capillary blood

- Ensure hands are clean. Avoid the use of wet wipes or alcohol wipes as these may affect the results.
- If hands are cold use warm water to wash with.
- Prick the side of fingers, avoiding the finger tips as this is a more sensitive area and frequent pricking may impair touch sensation.
- Use a different finger each time and avoid areas close to the nail bed.
- If insufficient blood hold the hand down allowing more blood flow to the fingers.
- Use the drop of capillary blood as indicated by the meter instructions.
- Record the result.

Choice of blood glucose meter

It is important for patients to discuss their choice of BG meter with a member of the diabetes team to ensure they have the meter that is most appropriate for their needs. There are several available on the market, all of which have aimed to reduce the margins for error, such as those that require no calibration or coding.

Cleaning and checking the accuracy of blood glucose meters

In order to check the accuracy of home estimated BG measurements it is important that:

- The meter is maintained as per the manufacturer's instructions, and coded and calibrated with the test strips if necessary.
- Blood glucose monitoring strips are in date and have been stored according to manufacturer's instructions.
- Test solutions of a known glucose value are be used to check the accuracy of the meter.

Using blood glucose monitoring cost effectively

Blood glucose monitoring test strips are expensive and account for the largest part of the cost of managing diabetes. Several primary care trusts have recently instructed primary care staff to reduce provision of BG monitoring test strips to individuals with diabetes, particularly those with Type 2 diabetes who are on diet and/or metformin and/or glitazones alone. (See 📖 Blood glucose monitoring and types of diabetes, p. 94, regarding timing and frequency.)

Blood glucose monitoring and types of diabetes

Type 1 diabetes

Blood glucose monitoring is seen as an integral part of managing Type 1 diabetes patients, the majority of whom will be on basal bolus therapy. Individuals with Type 1 diabetes as part of structured education programmes will learn how to monitor BG control and adjust insulin therapy accordingly. This will include both pre- and post-prandial (after meal) testing. People with Type 1 diabetes are more liable to instability of BG control and so monitoring BG levels should ideally take place at least 4 times per day. Factors that require more frequent testing include:

• Hypoglycaemic unawareness.
• Frequent hypoglycaemia.
• Exercise.
• Inter-current illness.
• Pregnancy.
• Breast feeding.
• Driving.
• Certain employments.
• Drug and alcohol abuse.
• Change of insulin regimes.
• Advanced complications.

Type 2 diabetes

As in Type 1 diabetes, BG monitoring should form part of an integral self-management programme, although individuals with Type 2 diabetes are less prone to the extremes of BG levels found in Type 1.

The insulin regime and goals of therapy should determine the frequency and timing of BG monitoring. Some individuals on basal insulin only may only test fasting BG levels.

Those on twice daily pre-mixed insulin are recommended to monitor twice daily at various pre- and post-prandial (after meal) times and before bed. This will enable the individual to determine trends and consistencies in results, and adjust insulin doses appropriately. If on basal bolus (MDI) insulin therapy, they should monitor with the same frequency as in Type 1 diabetes.

Oral treatment

For those individuals who are not on sulphonylureas or secretagogues, such as meglitinides, where there is no risk of hypoglycaemia, self-monitoring of BG may be beneficial if the individual is going to use the results to modify self-care behaviour, such as diet and exercise. This information may help motivate individuals to improve their diabetes control.

Those on sulphonylureas and post-prandial regulators, where there is a risk of hypoglycaemia, may wish to monitor at variable times of the day to assess BG control, and at times when risk of hypoglycaemia is greater, i.e. during exercise.

Blood glucose monitoring is a valuable tool for individuals with Type 1 and Type 2 diabetes. It facilitates patient empowerment if the individual has the knowledge, skills, and confidence to adjust their diabetes treatment to achieve satisfactory glycaemic control. Structured education should enable the individual achieve this, without inappropriate over-use of test strips.

Blood testing for ketones

Some BG meters also have the ability to test for blood ketones, utilizing blood ketone test strips (see 📖 Urine test results: ketones, p. 136).

Further information

Owens D, Barnett AH, Pickup J et al (2004). Blood glucose monitoring in Type 1 and Type 2 diabetes: reaching a multidisciplinary consensus. *Diabetes Primary Care* **6**, 8–16.

Assessing blood glucose control

There is little point in obtaining BG results if action regarding treatment is indicated, but none is taken. Individuals need to be clear:

- When it is appropriate to test.
- How often.
- What the target BG level should be and how this may be achieved.

If results fall outside of agreed target range an assessment will need to be carried out to try and identify the potential cause(s) of the deterioration in control. These may include (see Table 5.1):

- Diet, too much CHO, or inclusion of refined CHO in diet, over compensation in the treatment of hypoglycaemia or caution to prevent hypoglycaemia.
- Infection/illness, any symptoms of infection, raised temperature, raised WCC/ESR.
- Stress, any recent stress in the short- or long-term.
- Reduced activity.
- Drug-induced? Any recent introduction of medications that may cause hyperglycaemia, e.g. steroids.
- Counter-regulatory hormone excess, in response to hypoglycaemia, or counter-regulatory hormones, during illness, are raised.
- Treatment related? Taking oral hypoglycaemic agents, time taken in relation to meals.
- Treatment related, for those individuals on insulin, poor absorption, due to problems with injection sites, timing of insulin inappropriate in relation to meal, inappropriate self-adjustment of insulin, insulin pen failure.
- Insulin past expiry date, or ineffective if incorrect storage and exposure to extremes of temperature.

If hypoglycaemia is experienced on a regular basis, treatment may also need to be adjusted (see Chapter 8, pp. 161–178).

Table 5.1 Assessing blood glucose control

Causes of raised BG levels	Causes of low BG levels
Increase in CHO intake	Decrease or insufficient CHO intake
Reduced activity	Increased activity
Insufficient glucose lowering medication, oral agents and/or insulin, or poor compliance	Dose of glucose lowering medication, oral agents and/or insulin too high
Insulin-related, poor technique, insulin out of date	Alcohol
Infection, illness stress	Weight loss causing insulin and/or oral agents to be more effective
Medication introduced	Deterioration in renal function
Rebound hyperglycaemia following hypoglycaemia	

(See 📖 Hyperglycaemia, p. 168; 📖 Hypoglycaemia: overview and symptoms, 162)

References

Elschen LMC, Bloemendal E, Nijpels G, et al (2007) Self-monitoring of blood glucose in patients with type 2 diabetes mellitus who are not using insulin. *Cochrane Database of Systematic Reviews.* Issue 4.

Hussein SF, Siddique H, Coates P, Green J. (2007) Lipoatrophy a thing of the past, or is it? *Diabet Med* **24**, 1470–2.

Self-adjustment of insulin

Self-adjustment of insulin is preferable for those patients taking insulin; this allows the individual more control and flexibility in their diabetes management.

Insulin may need to be increased in the following circumstances

- Increased CHO intake.
- Blood glucose levels outside of target range.
- Illness.
- If medications are commenced that are hyperglycaemic, e.g. steroids.
- Stress.
- Reduced activity.

Insulin may need to be decreased in the following circumstances

- Reduced food intake.
- Repeated episodes of hypoglycaemia.
- Increased activity.

The insulin regime used and BG profiles will determine which insulin dose will need adjusting. Alongside this the individual's target BG levels and target HbA1c will also determine how aggressive the insulin adjustment needs to be.

General principles include:
- Consider adjusting one dose at a time.
- Consider a percentage increase of total dose. In order for an insulin adjustment to be effective, a 10% increase or decrease is suggested, e.g. increase of 2units on a 20 total dose = 10%. Increase of 2units on a 50u total dose = <5% and is unlikely to be effective.
- Encourage individuals to be proactive, rather than reactive, i.e. anticipating an increase in CHO, rather than taking extra insulin after the event.
- In structured education programmes for people with Type 1 diabetes meal time insulin is calculated according to CHO intake, the same as it is for pump therapy (see 📖 Commencing pump therapy, p. 90).

Examples of blood glucose profiles that require insulin adjustment

Table 5.2 Regimen BD analogue mixture 22units am/20units pm

Pre-breakfast	Post-breakfast	Pre-lunch	Post-lunch	Pre-evening meal	Post-evening meal	Before bed
11.9	8.0	5.6	8.7	4.9	13.0	16.7
12.7		4.3			11.9	15.9
13	9.0	6.0		5.4	10.9	14.0

1 Suggested adjustment, based on post-evening meal, before bed, and fasting BG levels, increase p.m. insulin by 2 units, initially monitor response if no improvement in the following 2 days readings increase by further 2units (Table 5.2).

Table 5.3 Regimen once daily isophane insulin given nocte 40units

Pre-breakfast	Post-breakfast	Pre-lunch	Post-lunch	Pre-evening meal	Post-evening meal	Before bed
9.9	7.0					
8.7						
10.3			6.7			

2 Suggested adjustment based on fasting BG levels, increase insulin by 4u, monitor response if no improvements in the following 2 days increase by further 4units (Table 5.3).

Table 5.4 Regimen basal bolus regime nocte basal analogue 26units and tds analogue rapid-acting according to CHO intake

Pre-breakfast	Post-breakfast	Pre-lunch	Post-lunch	Pre-evening meal	Post-evening meal	Before bed
4.5	86	4.3	8.9	4.2	9.9	9.0
5.0		4.0			10.1	10.7
4.9	7.8	5.1		5.4	9.3	11.0

3 Suggested adjustment based on post-evening meal BG levels suggest insufficient insulin for CHO intake with evening meal (Table 5.4).

Table 5.5 Regimen basal bolus regime nocte basal analogue 34units and tds analogue rapid-acting according to CHO intake.

Pre-breakfast	Post-breakfast	Pre-lunch	Post-lunch	Pre-evening meal	Post-evening meal	Before bed
6.0	7.7	4.3	8.9	4.2	8.9	9.7
5.8		3.0			12.0	11.9
3.7	2.7	4.3		12.0	9.3	11.0

4 Suggested adjustment based on post breakfast and pre lunch BG levels suggest too much insulin for CHO intake with breakfast (Table 5.5).

Self-management: medication

The Department of Health *Management of Medicines* report stresses the importance of achieving tight glycaemic and bp control for people with Type 1 and Type 2 diabetes. However, it has been found that up to two-thirds of those prescribed oral hypoglycaemic medications do not take their tablets as prescribed (Donnan et al, 2002). Alongside this, most are unaware of any side effects that they might expect (Browne et al, 2000).

Of the 70% of people with Type 2 diabetes many take medications including:
- Oral hypoglycaemics.
- Insulin.
- Three or more hypertensives.
- Lipid lowering medication.
- Aspirin.

People with Type 2 diabetes take significant numbers of tablets. It is essential to ensure the patient understands the following:
- The action of medications.
- The correct dose.
- When to take the medication.
- The correct frequency and timing of dose each day.
- Possible side effects.

Because of the propensity for confusion caused by the numbers of pre-scribed medications it is important to review all the current medications they are taking:
- Those that are prescribed, Type dose regimen, contraindications.
- Those purchased over the counter (OTC).
- Any they may share with or have borrowed from others.
- Any family/homely natural remedies they may take.
- Any supplements.

Suggested questions to ascertain current medication taking behaviour

- How long have you been taking/using this medication?
- Is the medicine in its original container?
- Why do you take the medicine? What is its purpose?
- How often do you take it?
- Do you have a routine for taking it?
- Have you noticed any side effects since you have been taking it?
- Do you have any allergies to any medications?
- Do you take any medicines that have not been prescribed, but have been bought from the Internet, a chemist, shop, or supermarket, or when abroad?
- Has anyone lent you a medicine that is prescribed for them or which they have bought?
- Do you take any vitamin, supplements, herbal products, or homely remedies?
- Do you take any other forms of treatment/medication?

Further information

Diabetes National Service Framework ⊠ http://www.dh.gov.uk/PolicyandGuidance/HealthAndSocialCareTopics/Diabetes/fs/en

Browne DL, Avery L, Turner BC, Kerr D, Cavan DA. (2000) What do patients with diabetes know about their tablets? *Diabet Med*; **17**: 528–31.

Department of Health (2001) *National Service Framework for Diabetes Standards*. HMSO, London.

Department of Health (2001) *The expert patient: a new approach to chronic disease management in the 21st century*. HMSO, London.

Donnan PT, MacDonald TM, Morris AD. (2002) Adherence to prescribed oral hypoglycaemic medication in a population of patients with Type 2 diabetes: a retrospective cohort study. *Diabet Med* **19**(4), 279–84.

Urine testing

Glucose

Urine testing for glucose is relatively simple, and cheap in comparison to self-monitoring BG; however, there are some disadvantages.
These include:
- It is less sensitive than BG testing and is unable to detect hypoglycaemia.
- It is reliant on the renal threshold. The renal threshold is the level at which glucose overflows into the urine. The usual level for adults is 10mmol/l, although this can be variable. In elderly patients the threshold maybe higher, while in pregnancy it is often lower.
- Urine testing can only ever be a retrospective assessment of bloods glucose levels, as urine testing can only reflect BG levels since the bladder was last emptied.
- It is difficult to correlate urine glucose levels to BG levels.

If urine testing for glucose is carried out the patient will need to pass urine onto a reagent stick and then compare the colour change on the stick with the chart provided by the manufacturer.

To ensure accurate urine testing for glucose the individual should be advised to double void, i.e. empty the bladder and retest a new sample 30min later. If urine testing is considered to be the most appropriate for the individual, the test should be carried out on pre-breakfast samples and 2h after meals occasionally. The results should be used as a guide only and used in conjunction with an HbA1c result to determine overall diabetes control.

Ketones

Ketonuria is an indication of insufficient insulin to meet the bodies' requirements. This occurs in newly diagnosed Type 1 diabetes, and also during inter-current illness, when counter-regulatory hormones tend to be higher and there is insufficient insulin taken. Therefore, clinical indications for testing the urine for ketones include:
- If Type 1 diabetes is suspected.
- For the individuals with Type 1 diabetes during inter-current illness.
- For Type 2 patients on insulin, with a low BMI, who may be insulin depleted and therefore at risk of ketosis.

Performing the test is simple – the individual passes urine onto a reagent strip and the colour change on the stick is compared with a colour chart provided by the manufacturer. The degree of ketonuria is determined by the significance of the colour change.

If positive, an increase in insulin is indicated. The level of ketonuria will determine the urgency of an increase of insulin to prevent the development of diabetic ketoacidosis. If the result is significantly positive (see Urine test results: ketones, p. 136) during inter-current illness, urine should be tested for ketones at least twice a day until resolved. Alongside increasing insulin, increasing fluid intake will also facilitate the reduction of ketonuria.

Chapter 6

Self-management of diabetes

Structured education: meeting NICE criteria

Diabetes is a chronic condition and it is important that the person with diabetes becomes the expert in their own care. The aim of patient education is for people with diabetes to increase their knowledge skills and confidence, in order that they can take control of their diabetes and incorporate diabetes self-management into their daily lives. It has been demonstrated that structured education can improve biomedical outcomes and, therefore, reduce the risks of long-term complications, alongside improving the quality of life.

The NICE technology appraisal 60 *Guidance on the use of patient education models for diabetes* published in 2003 recommended that:

> Structured education is made available to all people with diabetes at the time of the initial diagnosis and then as required on an ongoing basis, based on a formal, regular assessment of need.

Whilst the guidance did not define the methodology or frequency of education sessions, the report suggested the education should reflect principles of adult learning, using a variety of teaching methods to promote active learning, engaging the participants as much as possible. These sessions should be provided by trained multidisciplinary teams and should be made accessible to the widest range of people with diabetes possible, taking into account cultural, geographical, and disability issues.

Diabetes UK and the Department of Health clarified further the requirements of structured education in the report from the Patient Education Working Group (2005) The key criteria agreed by the group included the following:
• A structured curriculum.
• Delivered by trained educators.
• Be quality assured.
• Be audited.

The structured curriculum must incorporate the following;
• A philosophy of supporting self-management attitudes, beliefs, knowledge, and skills.
• Be person centred, incorporating an assessment of the individual learning needs.
• Be reliable, valid, relevant, and comprehensive.
• Flexible and able to cope with diversity.
• Be able to incorporate different teaching methods.
• Be resource effective and have supporting materials.
• Be recognized as evolving based on new and emerging evidence.
• Must be written down.

Trained educators
- Need to have an understanding of education theory appropriate to the age and needs of the individual with diabetes.
- Be competent in the delivery of the educational theory of the programme they are offering.
- Be competent in the delivery of the principles and content of the specific programme they are offering.

Quality Assurance is essential to ensure the quality and validity of the structured education programme. Typically, programmes are peer reviewed internally and by external assessors. There are 3 main elements to the quality assurance process:
- Development of a defined programme, with a clear content, structure, curriculum, and underlying philosophy, which educators are trained to deliver.
- Defined quality assurance tools that define the observable core sets of behaviours required to deliver the programme.
- Internal and external process in place to assess the delivery and organization of the programme itself.

Audit the outcomes
Outcome data may include:
- Biomedical parameters.
- Quality of life measures.

In Type 1 diabetes DAFNE (Dose Adjustment For Normal Eating) is recognized as fulfilling the necessary criteria in structured education, although a number of locally developed programmes have been developed.

In Type 2 diabetes DESMOND (Diabetes Education for Self-Management Ongoing and Newly Diagnosed) and X-PERT meet the criteria.

Further information
Dose Adjustment For Normal Eating (DAFNE) ⊞ http://www.dafne.uk.com
Diabetes Education and Self Management for Ongoing and Newly Diagnosed (DESMOND) ⊞ www.desmond-project.org.uk
The X-PERT Programme ⊞ www.xpert-diabetes.org.uk

Effective consultations

In a long-term condition such as diabetes, consultations provide an opportunity for education, as well as assessing and addressing biomedical needs. A good consultation should primarily reflect the patient's agenda, rather than the health care professional's agenda, and should incorporate the following principles:

- Be based on empowerment philosophy.
- Promote understanding of diabetes and health risks.
- Promote intrinsic motivation to engage diabetes and self-management.
- Provide behavioural strategies and/or skills training.

Consultation skills

The start of the consultation will often set the tone for the remainder of the consultation; it is useful to start with an open question that facilitates the patient expressing their experiences and encourages them to tell you how they have been since their last visit. This should be followed by the patient being given the opportunity to express the topics or concerns they wish to address during the consultation; this enables the patient's agenda to be identified early on in the consultation:

- **Active listening:** when the consultation is underway, active listening is crucial. This can be demonstrated by asking open questions to seek clarity.
- **Paraphrasing the conversation:** this enables the health care professional to check that they have heard correctly and understood what has been said.
- **Acknowledging feelings:** feelings expressed during consultations can vary enormously from anger and frustration to distress. These can be expressed verbally or non-verbally. Ignoring feelings or emotions can potentially exacerbate them for patients.
- **Summarizing and ending the consultation:** it is essential to summarize the consultation prior to the end of the consultation. This enables the health care professional to clarify the content and feelings acknowledged. Ending the consultation should include goal setting and plans for follow up (Walker, 2000).

In summary, in order for consultations to be effective they need to include:

- An assessment of the individual's beliefs, behaviour, and knowledge.
- Provide information and benefits of behaviour change.
- Collaborative goal setting, and a discussion around ability and confidence to change behaviour.
- Barriers to self-care and/or behaviour change.
- Plan for follow up (Fig. 6.1).

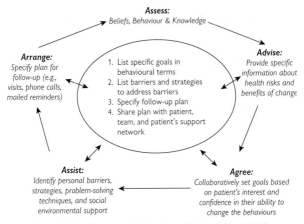

Fig. 6.1 The 5 A's for effective consultations. From Glasgow RE et al (2006) Assessing delivery of the five 'A's for patient-centered counseling. *Health Promotion International* **21**, 245–255, by permission of Oxford University Press.

Further information

Glasgow RE, Ermount S, Miller DC. (2006) Assessing delivery of the 5 A's of patient centered counseling. *Health Prom Internat* **21**, 245–53.
Walker R. (2000) Consultation skills: making a world of difference. *Diabetes Primary Care* **2**, 59–63.

Addressing the patient's agenda

Standard 3 of the National Service Framework (NSF) for Diabetes is entitled *Empowering people with diabetes* (Department of Health, 1999). The stated aim of this standard is to ensure that patients 'enhance their personal control over the day to day management of their diabetes'.

To achieve these aims, it is important to give people with diabetes time and attention when they voice their concerns and queries regarding their treatment prognosis and quality of life.

The Expert Patient Taskforce (Department of Health, 2001) noted a core of information required by people with diabetes to enable them to assert control over their lives:
- Knowing how to recognize and act upon symptoms.
- Dealing with acute attacks and exacerbation of their condition.
- How to use medicines and treatments effectively.
- Understanding the implications of professional advice.
- How to establish a stable pattern of sleep rest and deal with fatigue.
- How to access social and other services.
- How to manage work and the resources of the employment services.
- Knowledge and understanding of the consequences of different choices and actions.

There is a wealth of evidence to show the importance of achieving concordance with a patient regarding their agenda and treatment.

It is important to demonstrate respect for each patient – their views, cultural moirés and wishes – and to consider the way in which we communicate with patients at every consultation.

Identifying the patients' agenda at the beginning of the consultation will often set the tone for the remainder of the consultation. Asking open ended questions will help establish the patients agenda:
- What would you like to discuss today?
- Do you have any concerns you would like to raise today?
- What do you hope to get out of today's consultation?

Further information

Department of Health (1999) *Empowering people with diabetes.* National Service Framework, London.

Department of Health (2001) *The expert patient: a new approach to chronic disease management in the 21st century.* HMSO, London.

Health behaviour models

The diagnosis of diabetes requires the individual to make changes to diet and lifestyle. Behaviour change is a complex process, often difficult to achieve and sustain. In order to encourage healthy behaviours, health care professionals need to recognize many social, psychological, and environmental factors that influence the individuals' ability to make behaviour changes.

Health care beliefs

The health belief model is one of the first behaviour change theories developed. According to this model, changes in behaviour depend on five factors:
- **Perceived severity:** the belief that a health problem is serious.
- **Perceived threat:** the belief that one is susceptible to the problem.
- **Perceived benefit:** that changing ones behaviour will reduce the threat.
- **Perceived barriers:** a perception of the obstacles to changing ones behaviour.
- **Self-efficacy**: that one has the ability to change ones behaviour.

Example: A routine visit to the practice nurse reveals that a male patient is at risk of Type 2 diabetes due to a family history and obesity (perceived threat). He recognizes that his father died of complications related to his diabetes (perceived severity). The practice nurse informs him that losing weight and regular exercise will reduce his risk (perceived benefit). The man recognizes that he will find it hard to diet and increase his exercise due to work commitments (perceived barriers). However, he is keen to reduce his risk and joins the gym at work, enabling him to exercise during the working day, this proves successful for him and he loses weight (self-efficacy); Rosenstock et al, 1988).

Stages of change model

The stages of change model provide a framework for explaining how change behaviour occurs (see Fig. 6.2). According to this model there are 5 stages of change:
- **Precontemplation:** not thinking about behaviour change.
- **Contemplation:** thinking about changing in the near future.
- **Decision:** making a plan to change behaviour.
- **Action:** implementing the plan to change behaviour.
- **Maintenance:** continuation of behaviour change.

The stages of change model views behaviour as a process in which individuals are at various stages of readiness to change. It is not a linear model – individuals may be at any point in the model and people may stay in the same stage for a long period.

This model can be useful in assessing where an individual is in relation to changing behaviour, e.g. setting goals with an individual when they are in the pre-contemplation stage is unlikely to have success (Prochaska & Diclemente, 1994).

Social cognitive theory

The social cognitive theory suggests that behaviour change is influenced by the environment, personal factors, and aspects of the behaviour itself. The theory explains the education process through a number of contexts:

- **Reinforcement:** this is either the positive or negative consequences of behaviour.
- **Behaviour capability:** in order for a change to take place, the individual needs to know what to do and how (knowledge and skills).
- **Expectancies:** the value the individual places on the result of the change, if the result is important to the person, the behaviour change is more likely to happen.
- **Self-efficacy:** the belief in the ability to successfully change ones behaviour.
- **Reciprocal determinism**: the dynamic relationship between the individual and environment, and social support.

Social cognitive theory enables the health care professional to understand the complex relationships between the individual and his/her environment, how actions and conditions reinforce or discourage change, and the importance of believing in and knowing how to change.

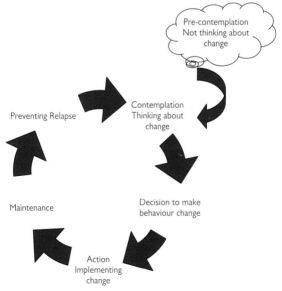

Fig. 6.2 Stages of change model (Prochaska & Diclemente, 1994).

Further information

Prochaska JO, Diclemente CC (1994). *Changing for good*. William Morrow, New York.
Rosenstock IM, Stecher VJ, Becker MH (1988). Social learning theory and the health belief model. *Health Education & Behaviour* **15**(2), 175–183.

Empowerment

The empowerment approach to diabetes education is intended to enable an individual to make informed decisions about their own diabetes care. Unlike the medical-centred model in which the health care professional is the expert, interview techniques are designed to reach a diagnosis and treatment is mainly the health care professionals' responsibility, and the individuals' role is to follow advice. The empowerment model recognizes that individuals control their treatment that the treatment is life long, that treatment involves aspects of daily living, treatment may affect quality of life, and ultimately individuals make choices the empowerment approach is more suited to chronic conditions and supports a patient centered model of care (see Table 6.1).

The empowerment approach consists of the following:
• Patient and professional agenda.
• Exploring the facts.
• Exploring thoughts and feelings.
• Professional honesty.
• Provision of options.
• Joint decision making.
• Joint action planning.

The empowerment approach requires the use of open-ended questions to:
• Discover what the individual thinks.
• Support their learning.
• To confirm theirs and your understanding.
• To show empathy and respect.
• To provide options and support decision-making.
• To turn decisions into actions.

It is worth reflecting on a recent consultation to establish what was said by the individual that confirmed their agenda was identified, the information was presented in a way they had requested, they understood what was being discussed, and that behaviour change was likely.

Table 6.1 Differences between medical centred model and patient centered model

Medical-centred model	Patient-centred model
Compliance	Autonomy
Adherence	Patient participation
Planning for patients	Planning with patients
Behaviour change	Empowerment
Passive patient	Active patient
Dependence	Independence
Health care professional determines needs	Patient defines needs

Further information

Skelton A. (2001) Evolution not revolution? The struggle for the recognition and development of patient education in the UK. *Patient Educat Counseling* **44**, 23–7.

Goal setting with patients

Diabetes often requires individuals to make lifestyle changes. In order to do this, individuals require a discussion around the options available, e.g. if an individual wants to lose weight, they may choose to eat less or exercise more. Initially, it is important to establish what the problem is, discuss potential solutions, evaluate these solutions for the individual, and then select the strategy to achieve the desired outcome.

Discuss what they are going to do and how; what are the barriers to achieving the goal and how will these be overcome; what support is available to help them achieve their goals. In order for goal setting to be successful a useful acronym to use is SMART:
• **S**pecific
• **M**easurable
• **A**ctions
• **R**ealistic
• **T**ime limited

e.g. 'I want to exercise more …'
• **Specific:** how much more?
• **Measurable:** how many days per week?
• **Action:** what will be done and when?
• **Realistic:** is this realistic?
• **Time limited:** when will this be achieved?

In order for goals to be achieved it is recommended that the patient leaves with an action plan that describes what they are going to do, considers the barriers to achieving this, and in what ways will the patient overcome these.

Confidence ruler

In order to establish success in achieving goals it is useful to assess the individuals' confidence in meeting a goal. This can be carried out by utilizing a confidence ruler:

1	2	3	4	5	6	7	8	9	10
Not confident									Very confident

Individuals are asked to circle the number that reflects their confidence to achieve a particular goal. A score of less than 5 demonstrates that it is unlikely that the goal will be achieved and suggests that an alternative goal/strategy should be considered.

Psychological aspects that influence self-management

Depression

Depression is a serious condition. It is 3 times more common in people with diabetes compared with the general population; it affects at least 15% of people with diabetes. Depression has a negative impact on self-management skills, including diet, blood glucose monitoring, and subsequently control. Ultimately, people with diabetes who are depressed are more likely to develop the long-term complications associated with diabetes (see 📖 Depression screening, p. 148).

Stress and anxiety

Stress and anxiety can cause an increase in the release of the counter-regulatory hormones that work in opposition to insulin – predominantly epinephrine and cortisol – when their production is increased. This is likely to increase blood glucose, and may cause or exacerbate hyperglycaemia.

The symptoms of anxiety, such as trembling, sweating, and palpitations, may also be confused with the symptoms of hypoglycaemia, leading to taking glucose unnecessarily and/or inappropriate adjustment of treatment.

The presence of stress and anxiety may also influence self-care behaviours, leading to episodes of poor blood glucose control.

Anger and frustration

The limitations diabetes imposes and subsequent additional self-care behaviours can lead to anger and frustration for the individual with diabetes.

Frequently individuals get frustrated when their blood glucose levels are difficult to control and this can lead to individuals 'giving up' managing their diabetes. As a result, they may eat inappropriately, miss tablets or injections, and fail to monitor blood glucose levels. This behaviour clearly exacerbates poor diabetes control.

Further information

Clark M. (2004) *Understanding diabetes.* John Wiley and Sons, Chichester.

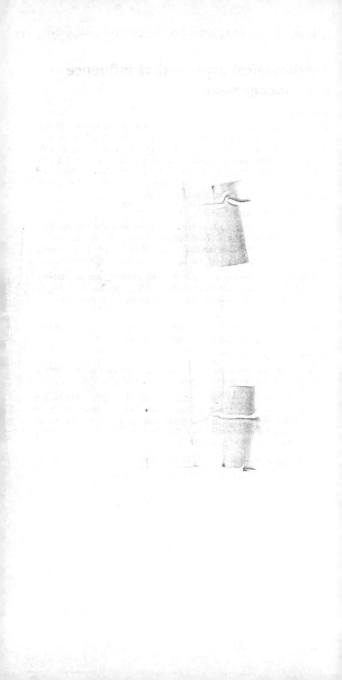

Monitoring diabetes

Annual review: interpreting results and target ranges

The annual review process

The Department of Health 2007 report by Sue Roberts (*Working together for better diabetes care: clinical case for change*) emphasizes the importance of offering patients annual review facilities at their general practice. This is more convenient for the patient and facilitates speedy referral by the GP of cases that need the attention of the specialist services clinic.

The purpose of the annual review is:
• To screen for complications.
• To identify risk factors.
• To assess educational needs.

The call and recall nature of annual review in primary care is predicated on the provision of a database of all patients with diabetes (as specified by the National Service Framework (NSF). It is therefore important that the following information is recorded:
• Name/date of birth/NHS number/date of next appointment.
• Type of diabetes and date of diagnosis:
  • Type 1
  • Type 2
  • Gestational diabetes
  • IGT
  • IFG.
• Height, weight, and BMI.
• Blood pressure.
• Latest blood results: HbA1c, serum creatinine, urea and electrolytes (U&E).
• Latest urine results: microalbuminurea.
• Peripheral pulses and sensation right/left normal/abnormal.
• Visual acuity right/left and retinal photo if available.
• Smoking status/education received.
• Seen by podiatrist, dietician, clinical nurse specialist, optometrist.
• Education received, diet, exercise, alcohol, monitoring.
• Treatment.

- Complications (date of onset):
  - angina
  - myocardial infarction (MI)
  - transient ischaemic attack (TIA)
  - peripheral vascular disease
  - retinopathy
  - neuropathy
  - foot ulcer
  - amputation
  - microalbuminurea
  - nephropathy.
- Procedures:
  - laser photocoagulation
  - coronary artery angioplasty
  - coronary artery bypass graft (CABG)
  - lower limb angioplasty or bypass
  - amputation
  - renal dialysis
  - renal transplant.

Further information

Roberts S. (2007). *Working together for better diabetes care.* Department of Health, London.

Screening for complications

A systematic enquiry regarding any symptoms the person with diabetes may have is required, including questions regarding:

- **Intermittent claudication:** does the person get muscular limb pain, usually in the leg, which is relieved by rest?
- **Angina:**
  - does the person have chest pain on exertion?
  - any other symptoms on exertion?
- **Erectile dysfunction:** sensitive questioning regarding sexual health and performance is required (see 📖 Chapter 10, pp. 219–232).
- **Neuropathic pain:** Does the person suffer from tingling, pain, or altered sensation in the feet? (see 📖 Foot assessment, p. 143).
- **Routine examination:** Undertake a routine examination of:
  - feet (see 📖 Foot assessment, p. 143)
  - fundoscopy with pupils dilated (see 📖 Visual acuity and retinal screening, p. 144)
  - blood pressure (see 📖 Blood pressure, p. 138).
- **Identifying risk factors – lifestyle:**
  - weight management/abdominal adiposity (see 📖 Waist circumference, p. 142)
  - exercise levels (see 📖 Exercise, p. 268)
  - smoking (see 📖 Smoking, p. 288)
  - family history of cardiovascular disease (CVD) and age of onset.
- **Identifying risk factors – laboratory test results**
  - HbA1c (see 📖 Blood test results: haemoglobin A1c, p. 124)
  - total cholesterol, triglycerides, high density lipoprotein (HDL), and low density lipoprotein (LDL) cholesterol (see 📖 Cholesterol, p. 130; 📖 Triglycerides, p. 132)
  - Creatinine (preferably U&Es as many patients should be on ACE inhibitors) (see 📖 Blood test results: urea and electrolytes, p. 126)
  - Lipids (see 📖 Blood test results: lipid profiles, p. 128)
  - Early morning urine albumin: creatinine ratio[1] (NICE guidelines for Type 2 assessment re ischaemic heart disease (IHD) (see 📖 Blood pressure, p. 138).

---

1 Urinary tract infections (UTIs) can give false positives.

Educational topics

It is important that the following areas are covered as part of a planned delivery of information to enable the person with diabetes to take an active part in the decision-making regarding their care:

- Monitoring/understanding risks and targets (see 📖 Annual review: interpreting results and target ranges, p. 120).
- Diet and maintenance of weight or weight loss (see 📖 Diet and diabetes, p. 70).
- Self-adjustment of medication (see 📖 Medication review, p. 156).

Further information

See also the recommendations of IDF (Europe) and Diabetes UK.

NICE (2002). CG87 *Type 2 Diabetes-newer agents: short guideline.* Available at 🖥 http://www.nice.org.uk/nicemedia/pdf/CG87Short Guideline.pdf (accessed 1st June 2009).

Blood test results: haemoglobin A1c

Haemoglobin A1c (HbA1c) or glycosylated HbA1c is a blood test to determine the amount of glucose in the circulating blood over time. The laboratory test is performed on a venous sample of blood and estimates the amount of glucose that has adhered to the haemoglobin in a red blood cell (erythrocyte). The higher the level of glucose in the circulating blood the more will stick to the haemoglobin and the higher the number in the HbA1c result.

Red blood cells are replaced in the circulation every 8–12 weeks and the HbA1c gives an estimation of the amount of circulating glucose over this time period. It is expressed as a percentage and an HbA1c of 4% would indicate that 4 in every 100 red blood cells had glucose attached to the haemoglobin.

It is used to monitor the long-term control of BG. Routine monitoring with HbA1c should be performed 6-monthly as a minimum, monitoring HbA1c more frequently in the following circumstances:
- Pregnancy.
- Following significant treatment changes, e.g. commencing insulin or an incretin mimetic.

Targets for people with Type 1 diabetes

The Diabetes Control and Complications Trial (DCCT Research Group 1993) established that maintaining HbA1c levels as close as possible to the normal range results in considerable reductions in long-term health complications, but it is worth noting this can be at the expense of hypoglycaemia, The patients achieving an HbA1c 7.2% in the DCCT experienced 3 times as many hypos:
- Normal range: 3.5–5.5%.
- NICE guidelines (2004) recommend a level of HbA1c below 7.5% to prevent the onset of microvascular disease and, in those at high risk of arterial disease, an HbA1c of 6.5% or below.

For people with Type 2 diabetes

The 1998 United Kingdom Prospective Diabetes Study (UKPDS) and the 2004 NICE guidelines for Type 2 diabetes indicate that glycaemic control is as important for people with Type 2 diabetes as for those with Type 1.

NICE has provided evidence statements to show that HbA1c estimates are predictors of macrovascular and microvascular complications, and that lowering the HbA1c lowers theses risks.

NICE recommend:
- HbA1c band of 6.5–7.5%.
- Based on the risk of macrovascular and microvascular complications for each patient (see 📖 Chapter 9, pp. 179–218).

Further information

DCCT Research Group (1993) The effect of intensive treatment of diabetes on the development and progression of long-term complications in insulin dependent diabetes mellitus. *N Engl J Med* **329**, 977–86.

NICE (2004) *Type 1 diabetes: diagnosis and management of Type 1 diabetes in adults.* NICE, London. Available at: ⊞ www.nice.org.uk (accessed 20th March 2008)

Blood test results: urea and electrolytes

Urea and electrolytes (U&E) are estimated in the laboratory from a venous blood test, which determines levels of:
- Sodium.
- Potassium.
- Chloride.
- Bicarbonate.
- Urea.
- Creatinine.

Sodium, potassium, chloride, and bicarbonate are dissolving salts and often referred to as electrolytes.

Urea is a product of protein breakdown, which is excreted through the kidneys. Creatinine is a product of the breakdown of creatinine phosphate required for the conservation of energy in muscle tissue.

The results are indicators of kidney function and therefore microvascular disease. If the kidneys are not working effectively the amount of urea and electrolytes found in the venous sample will be higher than the normal levels (Table 7.1).

Table 7.1 Normal levels

Urea	2.5–6.7mmol/l
Sodium	135–145mmol/l
Potassium	3.5–5.0mmol/l
Chloride	95–105mmol/l
Bicarbonate	24–30mmol/l
Creatinine	70–150µmol/l

The NSF for Renal Services (2006) recommends that for people with an increased risk of chronic kidney disease, an estimated glomerula filtration rate (eGFR) should be calculated and used as an indicator, instead of serum creatinine alone (Table 7.2).

This calculation by the laboratory uses a formula that utilizes the 4-variable modification of diet in renal disease (MDRD). The 4 variables are:
- Serum creatinine concentration.
- Patient's age.
- Patient's sex.
- Patients ethnic origin (for African-Caribbean people only, eGFR is multiplied by 1.21).

Table 7.2 Indications of the relationship between eGFR and the stages of kidney disease including frequency of retesting (⊟ www.dh. gov.uk/renal)

Stage of kidney disease	ml/min 1.73m²	Frequency of testing
1 Normal GFR[1]	>90	Annually
2 Mild Impairment[1]	60–80	Annually
3 Moderate impairment	30–59.6	Monthly
4 Severe impairment	15–29.3	Monthly
5 Established kidney disease	<15.3	Monthly

[1]The terms stage 1 and stage 2 chronic kidney disease are only applied when there is a structural abnormality that has been determined by ultrasound. For example, polycystic kidney disease or a functional abnormality, such as persistent protein urea or microscopic haematuria.

[2]If there is no such abnormality, a GFR of 60–89ml/min/1.73m is not regarded as abnormal.

Further information

Department of Health. Renal National Service Frameworks. ⊟ www.dh.gov.uk/renal.

Blood test results: lipid profile

Raised blood lipid levels (dyslipidaemia) are known to be a risk factor for coronary heart disease (CHD). A series of venous blood tests known as the lipid profile usually contain estimations of:
- Total cholesterol (TC), both HDL and LDL.
- Triglycerides.

In the UK, the average total cholesterol level is 5.7mmol/l.

NICE guidance on risk of coronary heart disease
Higher risk
- **Manifest cardiovascular disease (CVD):** a history or symptoms of:
  - coronary disease
  - stroke
  - peripheral vascular disease (PVD).
- With a 10-year coronary event risk assessed above 15%.

Lower risk
- No manifest CVD.
- A 10-year coronary event risk of 15% or below.
- Taking into account the limitations of the risk assessment charts.

Dyslipidaemia

This describes a group of conditions in which there are abnormal levels of lipids and lipoproteins circulating in the blood. People with either Type 1 or Type 2 diabetes may have dislipidaemia. However, people with Type 2 diabetes have hyperinsulinaemia, which can precipitate a reduced HDL cholesterol level and elevated triglyceride and LDL cholesterol levels.

Simply put, the core components of diabetic dislipidaemia are elevated circulating levels of triglycerides and LDL cholesterol, and decreased circulating levels of HDL cholesterol.

The NSF for CHD (Department of Health, 2000) recommends that serum total cholesterol should be reduced to below 5mmol/l and by at least 25% (serum LDL-cholesterol to below 3mmol/l and by at least 30%).

However, lower targets especially for secondary prevention and in diabetes and hypertension, e.g. European Atherosclerosis Society (EAS, 2002) recommend:
- Serum total cholesterol <4mmol/l.
- Serum LDL-cholesterol <2.6mmol/l.
- BHS serum total cholesterol <4mmol/l.
- Serum LDL-cholesterol <2.6mmol/l.

Also secondary targets are:
- Serum HDL-cholesterol >1mmol/l.
- Serum triglycerides <2.3mmol/l.

CVD accounts for 75% of deaths in people with Type 2 diabetes and 35% of people with Type 1 diabetes.

Comparing people with Type 1 and Type 2 diabetes, those with Type 1 have:
- 1/2 the rate of CHD.
- 1/3 rate of CVD.
- 2/3 rate of PVD.

However, the rates of all of these are greater than in those in the non-diabetic population.

Further information

Athyros VG, Mikhailidis DP, Papageorgiou AA, et al (2002) Attaining United Kingdom– European Atherosclerosis Society Low-density Lipoprotein Cholesterol Guideline target values in the Greek Atorvastatin and Coronary Heart Disease Evaluation (GREACE) Study. *Curr Med Res Opin* **18**, 499–502.

Department of Health (2000) *Coronary heart disease: national service framework for coronary heart disease – modern standards and service models.* Stationery Office, London.

Cholesterol

This is a body fat metabolized partly from ingested fats (about 30%) and mainly manufactured within the liver from saturated fats to produce low density lipoprotein (LDL) and high density lipoprotein (HDL) cholesterol.

Cholesterol is essential for cell structure, the production of some hormones, bile, and the protection of nerve cells. Cell membranes are dynamic structures that allow selective permeability for the transport of specific molecules from within the cell out and to allow other molecules to diffuse in. The lipid components of the cell membrane, phospholipids, glycolipids, and cholesterol form this permeable barrier.

Cholesterol is carried through the blood stream wrapped in lipoproteins. There are 5 kinds of lipoproteins:
- HDL.
- LDL.
- Very low density lipoproteins (VLDL).
- Intermediate density lipoproteins (IDL).
- Chylomicrons.

Due to their poor solubility in the blood stream, cholesterol, triglycerides, and other lipids require lipoprotein particles to act as transport vehicles. It is these transport vehicles that determine the 'good or bad' nature of cholesterol.

HDL cholesterol

Normally between 25 and 33% of total cholesterol is HDL, and it is referred to as 'good' cholesterol, as high levels of HDL have been shown to protect against heart disease. HDL cholesterol is also reported as having a beneficial effect on:
- Endothelial function.
- Leukocyte adhesion.
- Has an anti-oxidative effect.

More recently, it has been suggested that it has an effect on vascular structure and function, as it is thought to carry away excess cholesterol from the arteries and arterial plaques, to be processed in the liver.

Low levels of HDL cholesterol are seen to increase the risk of heart disease. HDL levels are assessed in relation to total cholesterol levels, the Joint British Society[1] Guidelines (2005) suggest an elevated total cholesterol to HDL ratio >6.0a is a risk factor for CVD.

LDL cholesterol

LDL contains more fat and less protein than HDL, and is less stable. LDL adheres to the walls of arteries and penetrates the protective inner lining of the endothelium Once cholesterol has migrated into the inner wall of the artery, it oxidizes and attracts triglycerides, sticky blood-clotting materials (e.g. fibrin and platelets) and white blood cells. Together, these substances form the building materials for plaque deposits, which are the hallmark of atherosclerosis.

This can lead to occlusion, and the formation of clots that can cause stroke and CHD. Clots and narrowing of blood vessels can occur in the legs causing reduced blood flow and pain, claudication, and an increase in the risk of foot problems (see 📖 Foot assessment, p. 143).

People with Type 2 diabetes have a tendency to produce small dense LDL cholesterol particles, which have a greater tendency to oxidize damage, rendering them even more atherogenic (prone to plaque production).

Further information

Joint British Society (2005) JBS guidelines on the prevention of CVD in clinical practice. *Heart* **91**(Suppl 5) 1–52.
(Joint British Society comprises British Cardiac Society, British Hypertension Society, Diabetes UK, HEART UK, Primary Care Cardiovascular Society, and the Stroke Association.)

Triglycerides

Triglycerides are major components of VLDL and chylomicrons, playing an important role in metabolism as energy sources and, along with cholesterol, as transporters of dietary fat. Triglycerides contain more than twice as much energy (9kcal/g) as carbohydrates and proteins.

The intestinal action (lipolysis) the combined action of lipases and bile secretions, splits triglycerides into glycerol and fatty acids.

Triglycerides are rebuilt in the blood from their fragments and become constituents of lipoproteins, which deliver the fatty acids to and from fat cells
- Tissues release the free fatty acids and take them up as a source of energy.
- Fat cells can synthesize and store triglycerides.

When the body requires fatty acids as an energy source, the hormone glucagon (see ⬚ Hypoglycaemia: treatment and consequences, p. 166) signals the breakdown of the triglycerides by hormone-sensitive lipase to release free fatty acids. As the brain can normally only use glucose as an energy source the liver can convert the glycerol component of triglycerides to glucose (gluoneogenesis).

High levels of triglycerides in the blood stream are linked to:
- Atherosclerosis.
- Increased risk of heart disease or stroke.
- Pancreatitis.

However, the negative impact of raised levels of triglycerides is lower than that of imbalance in the LDL:HDL ratios. The risk can be partly accounted for by a strong inverse relationship between triglyceride level and HDL-cholesterol level.

Although not measured in clinical practice there are 3 further types of cholesterol, which may become significant in the future.

Very low density lipoproteins

This very low density lipoprotein transports cholesterol and triglycerides within the body. It is created in the liver and contains the highest amount of triglyceride.

Intermediate density of lipoproteins

These are smaller and denser than VLDL. They are composed of 10–12% protein, 24–30% triglycerides, 25–27% phospholipids, 32–35% cholesteryl esters, and 8–10% cholesterol. IDLs are derived from triglyceride depletion of VLDL. IDLs can reprocessed by the liver or, upon further triglyceride depletion, become LDL.

Chylomicrons

These are the largest and the least dense of the lipoproteins. They contain 85–88% triglyceride, and transport dietary triglycerides and cholesterol, which has been absorbed by the intestinal epithelial cells.

NICE targets for reducing cholesterol

As a minimum, the target threshold for cholesterol should be reduction in TC to <5.0mmol/l or by 20–25%, whichever is the greater reduction, **or** Reduction in LDL-C to <3.0mmol/l or by 30%, whichever is the greater reduction.

Urine test results

Microalbuminuria

As serum creatinine is not sensitive to early kidney disease a urine test for microalbuminurea should be performed. Microalbuminuria is defined as a urinary albumin excretion rate of 30–300mg/day or 20–200μ/min.

Microalbuminuria offers the first sign of nephropathy occurring 5–15 years after the onset of Type 1 diabetes.

As people with Type 2 diabetes have often remained asymptomatic and unaware for some time microalbuminuria is often present at the time of diagnosis in Type 2 diabetes.

Associated with microalbuminuria are:
- Hypertension.
- A reduction in HDL cholesterol (see 📖 Cholesterol, p. 130).
- An increase in LDL cholesterol.
- An increase in triglycerides (fats which are present in blood plasma forming the plasma lipids in association with cholesterol) (see 📖 Triglycerides, p. 132).

Testing for microalbuminuria

It is important to check your local protocols/guidelines as there may be variations in different areas. If microalbuminurea is raised in an early morning urine specimen this is followed by the collection of a 24h specimen.

How to collect a 24h urine sample
- Urinate into the toilet first thing when rising on day 1.
- Then collect all the urine passed in the container(s) provided over the next 24h.
- Including the first urine passed on day 2.
- Cap the container and keep it in a cool place during the collection period.
- Make sure the container/s are labelled with:
  - the patient's name
  - the date of completing the test.
- Return the container as requested.

False positives for microalbuminuria can be caused by:
- Exercise.
- Urinary tract infection.
- Menstruation.
- Semen.

Risk factors for developing microalbuminuria:
- **Duration of the disease:** the longer a person has had diabetes the more likely there are to have microalbuminuria.
- Poor long-term glycaemic control (see 📖 Blood glucose monitoring: overview, p. 92).
- **Hypertension** (see 📖 Blood pressure, p. 138).
- **Dyslipidemia:** increase in LDL cholesterol and triglycerides and decrease in HDL cholesterol (see 📖 Cholesterol, p. 130; 📖 Triglycerides, p. 132).
- **Hyperfiltration:** symptomatic of early cardiac damage and/or metabolic syndrome (see 📖 Assessing cardiovascular risk, p. 158).
- Parents with renal disease.

Urine test results: ketones

Ketones (beta-hydroxybutyric acid, acetoacetic acid, and acetone) are the end-product of rapid or excessive fatty-acid breakdown. As is the case with glucose, ketones will be present in the urine when the blood levels of ketones surpass a certain threshold in the kidney.

Testing for ketones

This test is carried out using a dip stick, which changes colour depending on the amount of ketones present or may be tested with a blood ketone meter, which is more accurate but is not available in all areas.

The results are expressed as:
- **Neg.**
- **Trace:** 5mmg/dl.
- **Small:** 15mg/dl.
- **Moderate:** 40mg/dl.
- **Large:** 80–160mg/dl.

Blood ketone testing is also available.

Reasons for a positive test include:

Metabolic abnormalities
- **Uncontrolled diabetes:** diabetic ketoacidosis, a life-threatening event for people with Type 1 diabetes caused by absent or inadequate insulin levels.
- Glycogen storage disease.

Abnormal nutritional conditions
- Starvation or fasting.
- Anorexia.
- High protein or low carbohydrate diets.

Frequent vomiting
Hyperemesis gravis (a severe form of morning sickness in pregnancy).

Other disorders of increased metabolism, which may co-exist with diabetes and result in a positive test for urinary ketones
- Hyperthyroidism.
- Fever.
- Acute illness.
- Burns.
- Pregnancy.
- Lactation.
- Following surgery.

Blood pressure

People with diabetes have an increased risk of coronary heart disease (CHD) and stroke. 30–80% of those with Type 2 diabetes are hypertensive (raised bp; SHEP). The UKPDS has shown that controlling hypertension in people with Type 2 diabetes can reduce the risk of macrovascular and microvascular disease.

The hypertension optimal treatment (HOT) study 20 demonstrated that a diabetic cohort achieved a substantial reduction in cardiovascular (CV) events as a consequence of reduced bp (Hansson et al, 1998).

The 2004 NICE guidelines indicate the importance of hypertension control for people with Type 1 diabetes in order to reduce the risk of damage to their arteries.

The British Hypertension Society (BHS) suggests a bp of 130/85mmHg as the normal and recommends a threshold of above 140/90mmHg for initiating treatment for hypertension for people with Type 1 or Type 2 diabetes Their recommendation for target bp following treatment (both types of diabetes) is:
• 140/90mmHg.
• For those with nephropathy 130/80mmHg.
• For those with albuminuria 127/75mmHg.

The 2004 NICE guidelines recommend treating bp if:
• Above 135/85mmHg.
• Above 130/80mmHg if there is an abnormal albumin excretion rate or another symptom of metabolic syndrome:
  • higher waist circumference
  • low HDL cholesterol
  • high triglycerides.

See also 🕮 Waist circumference p. 142.

Although automated bp machines are used in many clinical areas, a paper by Matharu and Howell (2008) has shown that sometimes these can produce erroneous results. Bellamy et al (2008) recommend a mercury sphygmomanometer (spyg) as the best non-invasive method to use. Matharu and Howell note that it is therefore important to know how to use a mercury spyg correctly.

Taking blood pressure using a mercury sphygmomanometer

- Use a properly calibrated device that is regularly serviced and maintained.
- Routinely take the bp with the patient seated for at least 3 min.
- If the patient is an older person or someone with CVD, check bp with them standing.
- Remove restrictive clothing on the arm.
- Keep the arm supported at heart level and ensure the hand is relaxed.
- Ensure the cuff is of appropriate size.
- Inflate the cuff to 20–30mmHg above the loss of brachial pulse.
- Lower the column of mercury slowly (approx 2mm/s).
- With the eye level with the top of the mercury column read to the nearest 2mmHg.
- Measure diastolic at the disappearance of sound (phase v).
- Take the mean of at least 2 recordings. If a discrepancy above 5mmHg take additional readings.
- When estimating CV risk in diabetes, use an average of results over several visits to the surgery/clinic (adapted from the BHS guidelines).

Table 7.3 Blood pressure cuff sizes for mercury spyg, semi-automatic and ambulatory monitors (BHS recommendations)

Indication	Bladder width and length	Arm circumference
Small adult/child	12 × 18cm	<23cm
Standard adult	12 × 26cm	<33cm
Large adult	12 × 40cm	<50cm
Adult thigh cuff	20 × 42cm	<53cm

Further information

Bellamy JE, Pugh H, Sanders DJ (2008). The trouble with blood pressure cuffs. *BMJ* **337**: a431.

BHS Nurse Distance Learning Course. *Lets do it well.* Available at: 🖥 www.bhsoc.org/pdfs/hit.pdf (accessed 20 March 2009).

Hansson L, Zanchetti A, Carruthers SG, et al. (1998) Effects of intensive blood-pressure lowering and low-dose aspirin in patients with hypertension: principal results of the Hypertension Optimal Treatment (HOT) randomised trial. *Lancet* **351**,1755–62.

Matharu G, Howell S (2008). Hypertension or poor technique. *Student Br Med J.* Available at: 🖥 http://student.bmj.com/issues/08/09/education/322.php (accessed 2 October 2008).

Systolic Hypertension in the Elderly (SHEP) Co-operative Research Group.(1991) Prevention of stroke by antihypertensive drug treatment in older persons with isolated systolic hypertension: final results of the SHEP. *J Am Med Ass* **265**, 3255–64.

Body mass index

Body mass index is a method of finding if you are a healthy weight for your height, age, and frame. Using a BMI calculator (an example is available at NHS Direct: 🖳 www.nhsdirect.nhs.uk/interactivetools/bmi.aspx), enter current:
- Height and weight.
- Frame size – small, medium, or large frame.
- Male or female.

Body frame size is determined by a person's wrist circumference in relation to their height to determine body frame size (see Table 7.4).

The following weight ranges were set by the WHO:
- **BMI less than 18.4:** underweight for height.
- **BMI between 25 and 29.9:** ideal weight for height.
- **BMI between 30 and 39.9:** obese.
- **BMI over 40:** very obese.

However, BMI is not accurate if the patient is:
- A weight trainer.
- An athlete.
- Pregnant.
- Breastfeeding.
- Over 60 years of age.

About 80% of people who have Type 2 diabetes are overweight, and there is a relationship between the amount of deep abdominal visceral and upper body fat and insulin resistance, Type 2 diabetes, cardiovascular disease, and abnormal body fat levels. Central obesity has been associated with:
- Decreased glucose tolerance.
- Alterations in glucose insulin homeostasis.
- Reduced metabolic clearance of insulin.
- Decreased insulin-stimulated glucose disposal.

Insulin resistance and the resulting impaired glucose control form part of what is known as metabolic syndrome. One definition for this syndrome is if the patient has 3 or more of the following (National Cholesterol Education Programme):
- **Central obesity:** waist circumference – male >102cm, female >88cm.
- **Hypertriglyceridaemia:** triglycerides ≥1.7mmol/l.
- Low HDL:
  - <1.0mmol/l male;
  - <1.3mmol/l female.
- **Hypertension:** ≥135/85mmHg or on medication.
- **Fasting plasma glucose:** ≥6.1mmol/l.

NB. Not all people with metabolic syndrome will develop Type 2 diabetes, but it as a risk factor.

Further information

National Cholesterol Education Programme (2001) *Adult Treatment International Diabetes Panel.* NCEP: Amsterdam, The Netherlands.

Waist circumference

In 2005 the International Diabetes Federation delineated specific waist circumferences as indicators of central trunk obesity for different ethnic groupings.
- **Europeans:** male ≥94cm, female ≥80cm.
- **South Asians and Chinese:** male ≥90cm, female ≥80cm.
- **Japanese:** male ≥85cm, female ≥90cm.
- **Ethnic South and Central Americans:** as per South Asian (no current data).
- **Sub-Saharan African:** as per European (no current data).

It is important to consider BMI as a gauge for general obesity and waist circumference as a guide to abdominal visceral fat deposits. Waist circumference measures have been shown to be a better indictor of this than waist to hip ratio.

Table 7.4 Calculate body frame size for BMI estimation

Gender	Height	Wrist size	Frame
Women	under 5'2" (157cm)	Wrist size less than 5.5" (14cm)	Small
		5.5–5.75" (14–15cm)	Medium
		over 5.75" (15cm)	Large
	5'2" (157cm) to 5'5" (165cm)	Less than 6" (15cm)	Small
		6–6.25" (15–16cm)	Medium
		Over 6.5" (17cm)	Large
	Over 5'5" (165cm)	Less than 6.25" (16cm)	Small
		6.25–6.5" (16–17cm)	Medium
		Over 6.5" (17cm)	Large
Men	Over 5'5" (165cm)	5.5–6.5" (14–17cm)	Small
		6.5–7.5" (17–19cm)	Medium
		Over 7.5" (19cg)	Large

Further information

International Diabetes Federation (2005) *The IDF consensus worldwide definition of the metabolic syndrome.* Available at: ⌨ http://www.idf.org/webdata/docs/Metac_syndrome_def.pdf (accessed 29 January 2006).

Foot assessment

The NHS Diabetes Support Team documentation suggests that examination of the feet of a person with diabetes at annual review should include:

- Testing foot sensation using either:
  - a 10g monofilament
  - vibration.
- Palpation of foot pulses.
- Inspection of any foot deformity and foot wear.

A foot should be classified regarding foot ulceration as:

- At low current risk.
- At increased risk.
- At high risk.
- An ulcerated foot.

If the person is found to be at low current risk, a management plan including education should be agreed.

- If the person is found to be at increased risk, perhaps showing signs of neuropathy, absent pulses, or other risk factors, review 3–6-monthly:
  - inspect the person's feet.
  - consider the need for vascular assessment.
  - evaluate current usual footwear.
  - enhance any specific foot care education as necessary.
- If the person is found to be at high risk of foot ulcers with perhaps neuropathy, or absent pulses plus deformity, skin changes, or evidence of a previous ulcer, review 1–3-monthly:
  - inspect the person's feet.
  - consider the need for vascular assessment.
  - evaluate and ensure provision of:
  - intensified foot care education;
  - specialist foot wear and insoles;
  - skin and nail care.

Ensure special arrangements for those people with access and mobility needs.

Further information

National Diabetes Support Team (2006). *Diabetic Foot Guide*. NHS: London. Available at ⧉ http://www.diabetes.nhs.uk/downloads/NDST_Diabetic_Foot_Guide.pdf

Visual acuity and retinal screening

Diabetic retinopathy is the largest cause of blindness in the working population of the western world. Retinal screening and visual acuity testing is required for both people with Type 1 and Type 2 diabetes. 60% of those who have had Type 2 diabetes for more than 20 years have pre-proliferated retinopathy. People with either Type 1 or Type 2 diabetes require retinal screening at the time of diagnosis. Depending on what is found this should be repeated yearly or, if deterioration is observed, an earlier review of and referral to an ophthalmologist may be indicated.

Visual acuity

Visual acuity (VA) is carried out in order to assess the limits of visual perception. Using a Snellen chart in a well-lit area, place the patient, wearing their distance correction glasses, 6m from the chart. (see Fig. 7.1). Test each eye separately:

- Occlude the eye not being tested.
- Test with and without distance glasses.
- If the acuity is below 6/6/ correct for any refractive error using a pinhole.
- Begin at the top of the chart and read progressively down.
- Vision is expressed as a fraction:
  - distance from chart in metres/lowest line read;
  - *upper number* – distance from chart conventionally 6m;
  - *lower number* – the distance at which an individual with no refractive error should see the chart.

If the top line cannot be read at 6m, it is moved toward the patient 1m at a time. If the top line still cannot be read at 1m, the tester will check for:

- Counting fingers (CF).
- Hand movement (HM).
- Perception of light (PL).

If VA is worse with pinhole consider maculopathy as cause.

Fundoscopy or ophthalmoscopy

The NICE review of the evidence suggests that fundoscopy or opthalmoscopy are unreliable for use in a retinal screening review, with the sensitivity of both GP's and optometrists proving to be very low.

Slit lamp biomicroscopy

NICE suggest that properly trained individuals carrying out slit lamp biomicroscopes with dilated indirect ophthalmoscopy can achieve sensitivities similar to the use of digital retinal photography.

Further information

NICE (2008). *Type 1 diabetes in adults: full guideline.* NICE, London. ▣ http://www.nice.org.uk/Guidance/CG15/Guidance/pdf/English (accessed 15 April 2009).

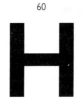

60

36

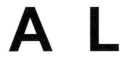

24

18

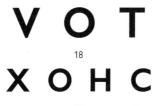

12

O H V C A

9

H A L C D X

6

V H A O X C T

5

Z H C X V O T A

4

H U O T X Z A V

Fig. 7.1 Snellen chart. Reproduced from Denniston A and Murray P (2006), *Oxford Handbook of Ophthalmology*, with permission from Oxford University Press.

Digital retinal photography

NICE found that digital retinal photography provided the highest level of accuracy of all screening methods.

NICE recommends yearly, or more frequently if necessary, assessment of the retina for people with both Type 1 and Type 2 diabetes, using retinal photography where possible.

Although there is some evidence to show that mydriasis (dilation of the pupil) may not be essential when using retinal photography, if more than one image is being taken it is essential. The NICE recommendations are to always use:

• Mydriasis (dilation of the pupil) using tropicamide 0.5% eye drops instilled into a pocket formed by pulling forward the lower lid is suitable for most patients.
• Patients should be warned that these eye drops may cause stinging for a few seconds following installation.
• Waiting with the eyes closed for a few minutes following instillation of the drops facilitates their absorption.
• Narrow angular glaucoma and previous eye surgery are contraindications.
• Reversal with pilocarpine is unnecessary and dangerous.
• Patients must be warned regarding blurred vision following the dilation affecting both their ability to drive and their motor insurance.
• Following the procedure, dark glasses may be useful if leaving the surgery/clinic in bright sunlight.

Further information

NICE (2008). *Type 1 diabetes in adults: full guideline*. NICE, London. ▣ http://www.nice.org.uk/Guidance/CG15/Guidance/pdf/English (accessed 15 April 2009).

Depression screening

Anderson et al's (2001) meta-analysis of depression rates found evidence that the odds for depression were twice as high in the group who had diabetes than a non-diabetic group. It has been suggested that depression is common in both people with Type 1 and Type 2 diabetes, and that it seriously affects the course and outcome of the disease.

The NICE guidelines suggest screening for depression using a recognized screening inventory, e.g. Beck Depression Inventory (BDI) or Hamilton rating scale for depression (HAMD).

Depression scales have groups of statements in the following areas:
- Sadness.
- Pessimism.
- Past failure.
- Loss of pleasure.
- Punishment feelings.
- Self-dislike.
- Self-criticism.
- Suicidal thoughts.
- Guilty feelings.
- Insomnia.
- Work problems.
- Slowness of thought reaction.
- Agitation/anxiety.
- Loss of appetite or weight without dieting.
- Sexual problems.

Using depression scales
- Patients are asked to choose one statement from each group.
- This should reflect how they have been feeling over the preceding fortnight.
- Each statement is given a numerical value, e.g. Feelings of Guilt section from the HAMD:
  - 0 = absent;
  - 1 = self-reproach, feel they let people down;
  - 2 = rumination over past errors sinful deeds;
  - 3 = present illness is a punishment, delusions of guilt;
  - 4 = hears accusatory or denunciatory voices and/or experiences threatening visual hallucinations.

- Each section carries a score; the totals are then matched against the scores:
  - **1–10:** these ups and downs are considered normal;
  - **11–16:** mild mood disturbance;
  - **17–20:** borderline clinical depression;
  - **21–30:** moderate depression;
  - **31–40:** severe depression;
  - **over 40:** extreme depression.

Even moderate depression can cause:
- Increased use of alcohol and tobacco.
- Reduction in quality of life and social functioning.
- Apathy leading to reduced physical activity.
- Reduction in motivation to follow recommendations in BG monitoring, insulin dose adjustment, diet, and exercise plan.

The Beck Depression Inventory is an example of validated questionnaire for assessing depression.

The following two questions are from the **Quality and Outcomes Framework** (QOF) and may be used to identify depression:
- During the last month, have you often been bothered by feeling down, depressed or hopeless?
- During the past month, have you often been bothered by having little interest or pleasure in doing things?

A yes response to either question is considered a positive result and is suggestive of depression; a no response to both questions makes depression highly unlikely.

Reviewing self-management skills: overview

Diabetes is a chronic condition and it is important that the person with diabetes becomes the expert in their own care. However, aspects of their self-management skills require review, as it is very easy to perpetuate sub-optimal practice. The annual review is an ideal time to look sensitively at areas of self-management and thereby to ensure best practice is being carried out.

Reviewing self-management skills

Injection sites

It is important to check:
- Injection sites.
- Rotation of injection within these sites to avoid diabetic lipodystrophies (see 📖 Chapter 5, pp. 81–104).

Further information

Hussein SF, Siddique H, Coates P, Green J. (2007) Lipoatrophy: a thing of the past, or is it? *Diabet Med* **24**, 1470–2.

Assessing patients' self-monitoring technique and results

Blood glucose

Research has shown that self-monitoring of BG is an important tool, both for improving glycaemic control, and in empowering people with Type 1 and Type 2 diabetes to be expert in managing their own condition (Welschen 2007). Irrespective of how long a person has been self-monitoring or how well they were taught, it is essential to check their BG estimation technique. As driving ability often deteriorates as we fall into bad habits through familiarity, so too the skill of BG estimation may become less than optimum.

The skill may be broken down into 4 main areas:
- Obtaining sample of capillary blood.
- Correctly using BG meter.
- Recording and interpreting results.
- Cleaning and checking accuracy of the BG meter.

Obtaining sample of capillary blood
- Wash and dry hands.
- Remind the person:
  - not to use wet wipes as they contain glycerin, which can affect the result.
  - avoid using scented or glycerol soap.
  - if hands are cold use warm water to wash with.
- Prick the side of fingers:
  - avoid using the finger tips as this is a more sensitive area and frequent pricking may impair touch sensation.
  - use a different finger each time and avoid areas close to the nail bed.
- If insufficient blood hold the hand down allowing more blood flow to the fingers.
- Use the drop of capillary blood as indicated by the meter instructions.
- Record the result.

Correctly using blood glucose meter
(see 📖 Blood glucose monitoring: overview, p. 92)

It is important for patients to discuss their choice of BG meter with a member of the diabetes team to ensure they have the meter that is most appropriate for their needs.

Recording and interpreting results

There is little point in obtaining BG results if action regarding treatment is indicated, but none is taken. Ensure patients are clear:
- When it is appropriate to test.
- How often.
- What the target BG level should be and how this may be achieved.

Cleaning and checking the accuracy of blood glucose meters

In order to check the accuracy of home-estimated BG measurements, it is important the meter is:
- Regularly cleaned and serviced, and test sticks are in date.
- Test solutions of a known glucose value are be used to check the accuracy of the meter.

Further information

Welschen LMC, Bloemendal E, Nijpels G, et al (2007) Self-monitoring of blood glucose in patients with Type 2 diabetes mellitus who are not using insulin. *Cochrane Database System Rev* **Issue 4**.

Urine testing: glucose

Urine testing for glucose is less sensitive than BG testing:
- The BG normally has to be above 10mm/l (the renal threshold) before glucose is present in the urine.
- Different people have different renal thresholds, which vary through life.
- It is difficult to be sure exactly what the relationship between glucose in the urine and BG is.

If urine testing for glucose is carried out, the patient will need to pass urine onto a reagent stick, then compare the colour change on the stick with the chart provided by the manufacturer.

If a pre-breakfast test is required, it is important that the person empties their bladder first and carries out the test on urine passed about 30min later.

Remind the patient to record the result immediately.

See also 📖 Urine test results: ketones, p. 136.

Evidence and subsequent treatment of hypoglycaemia

As we strive for tighter and tighter glycaemic control to reduce long-term complications, this lowering of BG will inevitably lead to an increased risk of hypoglycaemia (Wright et al 2006). Annual review gives an important chance to discuss the symptoms and treatment of hypoglycaemia with patients (see 📖 Hypoglycaemia: treatment and consequences, p. 166).

Signs and symptoms of hypoglycaemia will vary according to BG levels, duration of disease, alcohol intake, or frequent recent episodes of hypoglycaemia.

Hypos can be classified as:
• Mild (grade 1) where the patient can recognize and rectify them orally.
• Moderate (grade 2), which can be treated orally with the help of another person.
• Severe (grade 3), where the person is unconscious and unable to swallow.

It is also important to raise issues such as hypoglycaemia unawareness resulting from changes in the autonomic system.

Further information

Wright AD, Cull CA, Macleod KM, Holman RR, for the UKPDS Group. (2006) Hypoglycaemia in Type 2 diabetic patients randomized to and maintained on monotherapy with diet, sulfonylurea, metformin, or insulin for 6 years from diagnosis: UKPDS 73. *J Diabet Complicati* **20**, 402–8.

Medication review

The Department of Health *Management of Medicines* report stresses the importance of achieving tight glycaemic and bp control for people with Type 1 and Type 2 diabetes. However, it has been found that up to 2/3 of those prescribed oral hypoglycaemic medications do not take their tablets as prescribed (Donnan et al 2002).

That is:
- In relation to food.
- At the correct time.
- The correct dose.
- The correct frequency of dose each day.

Most are unaware of any side effects that they might expect (Brown et al 2000).

70% of people with Type 2 diabetes take many medications including:
- Oral hypoglycaemics.
- Insulin.
- Three or more hypertensives.

A further 30% of those with Type 2 diabetes have ischaemic heart disease and, therefore, also require:
- Lipid regulation medication.
- Aspirin.

Because of the propensity for confusion caused by the numbers of prescribed medications, it is important to ask patients attending annual review to bring with them all the current medications they are taking:
- Those that are prescribed.
- Those purchased over the counter (OTC).
- Any they may share with or have borrowed from others.
- Any family/homely natural remedies they make take.
- Any supplements.

These should be recorded and checked against those listed and expected.

A holistic review of the patient and their medication should be carried out checking for:
- Type.
- Dose.
- Regimen.
- Contraindications.
- Review of monitoring tests, e.g.
  - HbA1c
  - INR for those taking anticoagulants.

Types of questions that might be asked of a person with diabetes or their carer during their annual medication review

- How long have you been taking/using this medication/product?
- Is the medicine in its original container?
- Why do you take the medicine? What is its purpose?
- How often do you take it?
- Do you have a routine for taking it?
- Have you noticed any side effects since you have been taking it?
- Do you have any allergies to any medications?
- Do you take any medicines that have not been prescribed, but have been bought from the Internet, a chemist, a shop, or supermarket, or when abroad?
- Has anyone lent you a medicine that is prescribed for them or that they have bought?
- Do you take any vitamin, supplements, herbal products, or homely remedies?
- Do you take any other forms of treatment/medication?

Further information

Department of Health. Diabetes National Service Framework. 🖳 http://www.dh.gov.uk/PolicyandGuidance/HealthAndSocialCareTopics/Diabetes/fs/en (accessed 7th April 2009)

Browne DL, Avery L, Turner BC, et al (2000) What do patients with diabetes know about their tablets? *Diabet Med* **17**, 528–31.

Donnan PT, MacDonald TM, Morris AD. (2002) Adherence to prescribed oral hypoglycaemic medication in a population of patients with Type 2 diabetes: a retrospective cohort study. *Diabet Med.* **19**(4), 279–84.

Assessing cardiovascular risk

2008 RCT results regarding cardiovascular risk and treatment for Type 2 diabetes contrast with the findings of the UKPDS.

Action to Control Cardiovascular Risk in Diabetes (ACCORD) Trial

This trial randomized people with Type 2 diabetes into another intensive group, which targeted those with HbA1c of below 6% or a standard arm that targeted HbA1c results from 7–7.9%. It comprised:
- 10,251 people with Type 2 diabetes.
- With mean HBA1c of 8.1%.
- A mean age 62.2 years.

The primary outcome was a macrovascular composite of CVD death, or non-fatal stroke or myocardial infarct. More died in the intensive group so the trial was stopped after 3.5 years.

At 1 year the HBA1c was stable in the intensive group at 6.4% and in the standard group at 7.5%. During 3.5 years of follow-up the primary endpoint occurred in 352 people in the intensive group and 371 in the standard group, but 257 in the intensive group died compared with 203 in the standard group.

The Veterans Affairs Diabetes Trial (VADT):

VADT was a prospective, 2-armed, randomized control trial into independent cardiovascular (CV) outcomes for patients no longer responding to maximal doses of oral hypoglycaemics and/or insulin injections.

The population comprised:
- 1791 mostly male veterans.
- Veterans aged 41 and older.
- Veterans with Type 2 diabetes.
- Veterans enrolled over 2 years and followed-up for 5–7 years.

Results were presented at the 2008 Scientific Sessions of the American Diabetes Association (ADA). Findings showed AVANDIA(R) (rosiglitazone maleate), which was:
- Used in a majority of patients in the study.
- Was not associated with increased deaths.

However, the primary result of VADT did not show that intensive blood sugar control (HbA1c levels below 7%) had a statistically significant effect on reducing major CV events associated with diabetes.

Addressing the patient's agenda

Standard 3 of the NSF for Diabetes is entitled *Empowering people with diabetes*. The stated aim of this standard is to ensure that patients '*enhance their personal control over the day to day management of their diabetes*'.

To achieve these aims it is important to give people with diabetes time and attention when they voice their concerns and queries regarding their treatment prognosis and quality of life.

The Expert Patient Taskforce noted a core of information required by people with diabetes to enable them to assert control over their lives:
• Knowing how to recognize and act upon symptoms.
• Dealing with acute attacks and exacerbation of their condition.
• How to use medicines and treatments effectively.
• Understanding the implications of professional advice.
• How to establish a stable pattern of sleep rest and deal with fatigue.
• How to access social and other services.
• How to manage work and the resources of the employment services.
• Knowledge and understanding of the consequences of different choices and actions.

There is a wealth of evidence to show the importance of achieving concordance with a patient regarding their agenda and treatment. (see 📖 Goal setting with patients, p. 116)

It is important to demonstrate respect for each patient – their views, cultural moirés, and wishes – and to consider the way in which we communicate with patients at every consultation.

Smoking status

Smoking increases the risk factors for CVD and it is therefore essential to check this at annual review. For more information see 📖 Smoking, p. 288.

Alcohol intake

It is important to check that patients are aware of the Governments daily recommendations for alcohol intake of 2 units for women and 3 units for men. For more information see 📖 Alcohol, p. 284.

Further information

Department of Health (2001) *National Service Framework for Diabetes Standards*. HMSO, London.
Department of Health (2001) *The expert patient: a new approach to chronic disease management in the 21st century*. HMSO, London.

Chapter 8

Acute complications of diabetes

Hypoglycaemia: overview and symptoms

Hypoglycaemia: definition

Hypoglycaemia means low blood glucose (BG), clinically this would equate to BG less than 3.5mmol/l. To reduce the risk of hypoglycaemia individuals are advised to maintain a BG level over 4mmol/l.

Those at risk of hypoglycaemia are patients on insulin and sulphonylureas, those on diet alone, or diet and metformin are not at risk.

Physiology of hypoglycaemia

The brain is not able to store glucose so is reliant on a constant supply of glucose to function effectively. Any drop in BG levels below 3.5mmol/l will affect the central nervous system and impair cognitive function.

The normal physiological response to hypoglycaemia is the activation of both the autonomic and central nervous system:

- The release of counter-regulatory hormones, glucagon, and epinephrine occurs when BG levels drop between 3.6 and 3.8mmol/l.
- Autonomic symptoms occur when BG levels are ~3.2mmol/l.
- Cognitive function is affected generally when BG levels are <3.0mmol/l or less (see Fig. 8.1) the main symptoms of hypoglycaemia are related to the autonomic and adrenergic response or the neuroglycopenic effect.

Symptoms of hypoglycaemia

Autonomic symptoms: caused by epinephrine (adrenaline) production

- Trembling.
- Shaking.
- Anxiety.
- Sweating.
- Heart palpitations.
- Tingling lips.

Neuroglycopenic effect: deficiency of glucose to the brain

- Blurred or double vision.
- Headache.
- Slurred speech.
- Poor co-ordination.
- Unusual behaviour.
- Drowsiness.
- Confusion.
- Convulsions.
- Coma.

Whilst the clinical symptoms of hypoglycaemia are easily documented, the symptoms will vary between individuals and for the individual with diabetes may vary between hypos. The majority of patients learn to recognize their own symptoms. It is also possible for an individual to feel hypoglycaemic with normal BG levels. Typically, this would occur in an individual with long-standing poor control. When measures are put in place to improve BG control, people can feel hypoglycaemic as BG levels return to normal; the symptoms are caused by the drop and not by the actual BG level reached.

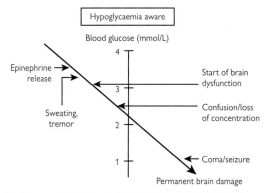

Fig. 8.1 Hypoglycaemia. Reproduced from Pickup J and Williams G (2004), *Handbook of Diabetes* 3rd edition, with permission from Wiley-Blackwell.

Reduced warnings for hypoglycaemia

There are a number of patients in whom warnings signs for hypoglycaemia have diminished, those individuals most at risk are:

• Those patients who have achieved near normoglycaemia.
• During pregnancy where glucose levels fall quicker in the fasting state.
• Concurrent medication, such as beta blockers, which prevent counter-regulatory response.
• Repeated episodes of hypoglycaemia causing diminished counter-regulatory hormone response.
• Long duration of Type 1 diabetes may also lead to lack of hypoglycaemic awareness.

Strategies to improve hypoglycaemia unawareness

• Strict avoidance of hypoglycaemia, this facilitates recovery of counter-regulatory response particularly adrenaline.
• Frequent BG monitoring and individualized training to increase awareness of glucose related symptoms.
• Individualized BG targets particularly for those patients at risk.
• Avoidance or moderation of alcohol, as alcohol reduces symptomatic awareness.
• Modification of insulin therapy as necessary.

Further information

Williams, G., Pickup, J. (2004) *Handbook of diabetes*, 3rd edn. Blackwell Science, Oxford.

Hypoglycaemia: causes

Potential common causes of hypoglycaemia
- Dietary.
- Diabetes medication related.
- Exercise/activity.
- Changes in other medication.
- Other medical conditions.

Dietary causes of hypoglycaemia
- Missing a meal.
- Delayed meal.
- Insufficient carbohydrate with a meal.
- Weight loss leading to increased sensitivity to insulin.
- Alcohol, as alcohol is metabolized in the liver the ability to release stores of glucose from the liver is compromised.
- Gastroparesis causing delayed digestion.

Diabetes medication related causes of hypoglycaemia
- Excessive or repeated doses of insulin.
- Honeymoon period post-diagnosis when beta cells partially recover and increase production of insulin.
- Deliberate overdose of insulin – suicide attempt.
- Dose of sulphonylurea too high.
- Poor injection sites leading to erratic absorption of insulin.
- Hot weather enhancing absorption of insulin.

Exercise/activity causes of hypoglycaemia
- Enhanced absorption of insulin.
- Increased insulin sensitivity.
- Insufficient carbohydrate pre-exercise and during exercise.
- Delayed hypoglycaemia secondary to muscles replacing glycogen stores.

Changes in other medications that may cause hypoglycaemia
Reduction of concurrent medication, such as steroids and thiazides, and some antipsychotic medications.

Other medical conditions that may cause hypoglycaemia
- Deteriorating renal function.
- Deteriorating liver function.

In the majority of cases the cause for hypoglycaemia can be identified, but replacement insulin therapy cannot match exactly the normal physiological production of endogenous insulin. As a result the risk of hypoglycaemia cannot be completely eliminated or a cause identified.

If the cause has been identified, education to prevent re-occurrence is necessary and a change in insulin therapy may also be indicated. Insulin analogues have been found to be useful to reduce hypoglycaemia, as has continuous infusion of insulin (see 📖 p. 88). In severe extreme cases islet cell transplant in Type 1 patients may be considered (see 📖 p. 313).

Hypoglycaemia: treatment and consequences

If possible confirming hypoglycaemia with a BG reading is recommended:

The aim of treating hypoglycaemia is to:
- Re-establish normal BG levels as soon as possible.
- Relieve symptoms.
- Identify cause to prevent re-occurrence and educate patient regarding future prevention.

Treatment examples following the 15/15/15 rule

- 15g of quick-acting carbohydrate, e.g. 80ml Lucozade, 5 glucose tablets, 5 jelly babies.

Followed by:
- 15g of long-acting carbohydrate, e.g. 2 plain biscuits, 1 slice of bread, or an apple.

Then patients should be advised to wait 15min and retest BG level. If the BG level has not returned to normal repeat above 2 steps.

Treatment for the unconscious patient

If the patient is unconscious and unable to swallow, do not give anything by mouth. A glucagon injection may be necessary. Glucagon® is the hormone made by the alpha cells in the pancreas; it raises BG levels by releasing stores of glucose from the liver (glycogen). A GlucaGen® kit is available on prescription. A glucogen injection will take approximately 15–20min to work, after which the patient is advised to take 15–20g carbohydrate orally. This may be administered by a relative/carer or, in some cases, paramedics will use GlucaGen® as first line treatment. Caution should be taken when using glucogen if the hypoglycaemic episode has been caused by alcohol as its effect may be significantly reduced.

Intravenous glucose remains the most rapid and effective treatment for severe hypoglycaemia. It is often the first line of treatment in most A&E departments and by paramedics. 50ml:50% dextrose is injected; this is best given in the antecubital vein to prevent thrombophlebitis and/or thrombosis.

It should be noted if the hypoglycaemia has been caused by sulphonylurea, the hypoglycaemic episode may last many hours, this requires regular monitoring of BG levels until normoglycaemia is achieved.

Consequences of hypoglycaemia

Physiological

- **Poor BG control:** a number of patients choose to run their BG levels high in order to prevent/avoid hypoglycaemia, but this will increase the risk of long-term complications.
- **Somogyi effect:** this describes the rebound high BG levels following a hypoglycaemic episode. This is predominantly related to the counter-regulatory response to hypoglycaemia and it can also be exacerbated by over treatment with oral glucose. The Somogyi effect is often recognized in the fasting BG level. This may be significantly raised and is caused by the patient experiencing nocturnal hypoglycaemia. Some patients may sleep through this and not necessarily have wakened. The counter-regulatory response will have been sufficient to correct the hypoglycaemia, resulting in a raised fasting BG level.
- **A direct relationship between hypoglycaemia and death** has been proposed, a very rare disorder characterized by an unexpected death in a previously healthy, tightly controlled Type 1 young person, often associated with a history of recurrent nocturnal hypoglycaemia. This syndrome is thought to be as a result of a fatal ventricular arrhythmia caused by hypoglycaemia – induced lengthening of the QT interval.
- **Hypoglycaemia** is also a potential cause of car accidents.

Psychological

Patients treated with insulin or sulphonylureas live under the constant threat of hypoglycaemia. It is a complication feared by both patients and health care professionals. Patients may become anxious to avoid hypogly-caemia, as it can lead to a feeling of loss of control and/or a behaviour change. This can also lead to a lack of self-confidence and a reduction in physical activity, as it is avoided in order to prevent hypoglycaemia.

Referral

If a patient is experiencing repeated episodes of recurrent hypoglycaemia, and no obvious causes have been identified or the problem remains unre-solved despite intervention, referral to a specialist team is recommended.

Hyperglycaemia

Can be described as high BG levels.

Definition

Normal BG levels range between 3.5–7.5mmol/l so by definition any BG level consistently above 7.5mmol/l is hyperglycaemia. However, the individuals' circumstances may influence the level as which hyperglycaemia is determined, for example, in pregnancy where strict BG control is essential, any levels beyond normoglycaemia require intervention. Typically BG levels greater than 10mmol/l would be defined as hyperglycaemia.

Symptoms of hyperglycaemia

- **Lethargy:** as energy source glucose not being utilized effectively.
- **Polyuria/nocturia** increased urine output secondary to osmolar diuresis.
- **Polydipsia, dry mouth:** a compensating symptom to prevent dehydration.
- **Cramp in legs:** muscles unable to access glucose.
- **Blurred vision:** changes in visual acuity caused by lens changing shape.
- **Abdominal pain**.
- **Weight loss** in some cases.

Causes of hyperglycaemia

Potential common causes of hyperglycaemia
- Dietary.
- Diabetes medication related.
- Exercise/activity.
- Changes in other medication.
- Other medical conditions.

Dietary causes of hyperglycaemia
- Excess carbohydrate with a meal.
- Excess refined carbohydrate.
- Weight gain leading to reduced sensitivity to insulin.

Diabetes medication related causes of hyper glycaemia
- Insufficient dose of insulin.
- Missed dose of insulin, either inadvertently or deliberately.
- Insulin degradation (inadvertent freezing, out of date).
- Insufficient treatments with oral hypoglycaemic agents.
- Poor injection sites leading to erratic absorption of insulin, e.g. hyperlipertrophy.
- Poor injection technique, insulin delivered intradermally.

Exercise/activity causes of hyperglycaemia
- Lack of exercise.
- Less exercise taken than planned.
- Excess carbohydrate pre-exercise.

Changes in other medications that may cause hyperglycaemia
Commencement of concurrent medication, such as steroids and thiazides, and some anti-psychotic medications.

Other medical conditions that may cause hyperglycaemia
- Acute illness.
- Infection.
- Menstrual cycle.
- Stress.

Treatment of hyperglycaemia

The treatment of hyperglycaemia will largely depend on the cause. If BG levels are consistently in the hyperglycaemic range, it will increase the risk of the long-term complications of diabetes and so will require intervention. Having identified the cause, the most appropriate treatment can be defined.

Principles of treatment
- Increase fluid intake or sugar-free fluids to prevent dehydration.
- Reducing refined carbohydrate intake.
- Reduce quantity of carbohydrate at each meal.
- Optimizing insulin treatment and ensuring doses are sufficient. Temporary increases in insulin may be necessary, and making sure that insulin is in date, has been stored appropriately, and ensuring injection sites are satisfactory.
- Optimizing oral hypoglycaemic treatment, consider concordance with treatment.
- Education regarding the benefits of exercise and appropriate planning for exercise. In the Type 1 patient exercise should be avoided if the BG level is above 15mmol.
- Treat any illness and infection promptly.
- Identify pattern of BG levels caused by new concomitant medication, and adjust hypoglycaemic treatment as necessary, both insulin and oral agents.
- Consider causes of stress and, where possible, help the patient to identify coping strategies.

Intercurrent illness and infections

Intercurrent illness can influence diabetes control dramatically. During illness, levels of the counter-regulatory hormones, epinephrine, glucagon, growth hormone, and cortisol all rise, the impact of these hormones particularly in the liver cause gluoconeogenisis, glycogen, and lipolysis (fat breakdown). In people with Type 1 diabetes, in whom the ability to produce insulin is absent, or in Type 2, where the ability to increase insulin production is reduced, this leads to hyperglycaemia.

Poorly controlled diabetes is associated with a wide range of infections, which tend to be more frequent than in the general population. These include:
- Urinary tract infections.
- Respiratory infections.
- Soft tissue infections.
- Dental infections/tooth decay.

Infections predominantly occurring in people with diabetes
- Malignant otitis externa.
- Rhinocerebral mucormycosis.
- Necrotizing fascilitis.
- Fournier's gangrene.
- Emphysematous infections.
- Emphysematous cholecystis.
- Emphysematous pyelonephritis, pyelitis, and cystisis.
- Infections in the diabetic foot.

(See Williams and Pickup, 2004.)

The increased susceptibility to infections is caused by:
- Impaired neutrophil/leukocyte function, chemotaxis, phagocytosis, and bactericidal activity, all of which will potentially reduce host defences against infection.
- *Staphylococcus aureus* skin transportation is more common in patients with Type 1 diabetes, leading to poor wound healing and soft tissue infection if trauma occurs.

Treatment

- Monitor BG levels frequently (at least 4 times/day), and optimize diabetes control, maintaining usual treatment. A temporary increase in insulin may be necessary or insulin may need to be commenced.
- **Insulin should never be stopped**, even if the patient is not eating or drinking.
- If unable to tolerate their usual food, the patient should be advised to maintain fluid intake and replace meals with fluids containing carbohydrate.
- In Type 1 diabetes, check for ketones and seek advice from the diabetes specialist team if positive.
- **Treat infection promptly:** where possible obtain sample for culture and specificity. Commence broad spectrum antibiotics as soon as possible until culture and sensitivity available.

Further information

Williams G, Pickup J. (2004) *Handbook of diabetes*, 3rd edn. Blackwell Science, Oxford.

Diabetic ketoacidosis

Diabetic ketoacidosis (DKA) is a serious acute complication of diabetes, occurring in patients with Type 1 diabetes or in Type 2 patients on insulin who are insulin-deficient, rather than insulin-resistant.

Physiology

Diabetic ketoacidosis occurs as a result of insulin deficiency and increased counter-regulatory hormones.

Insulin deficiency leads to:
- Increased hepatic glucose production.
- Increased gluconeogenesis.
- Reduced uptake of glucose into skeletal muscle and fat cells.

Counter-regulatory hormone excess in particular glucagon leads to:
- Hepatic gluconeogenesis contributing to hyperglycaemia.
- Stimulates release of free fatty acids into the circulation, where the liver synthesizes these into ketone bodies, acetoacetone, beta-hydroxybutyrate, and acetone.

Precipitating causes of diabetic ketoacidosis
- Infection.
- Acute illness.
- Errors in insulin management, i.e. insulin stopped inappropriately.
- New diagnosis of Type 1 diabetes.
- Deliberate omission of insulin.

Clinical features
- Polyuria, polydipsia, nocturia.
- Lethargy, weakness.
- Nausea and vomiting.
- Abdominal pain.
- Kussmaul respirations (laboured breathing).
- Altered level of consciousness.
- Hyperglycaemia.
- Ketonuria/ketonaemia.
- Smell of ketones (acetone on the breath).

The severity of the symptoms will depend on the severity of DKA.

A rapid assessment is required, a full clinical history must be taken. Investigations should include:
- BG level.
- Bicarbonate level.
- Urea and electrolytes.
- Blood gases.
- Full blood count to establish precipitating factors.
- Blood culture to establish precipitating factors.
- Chest X-ray to establish precipitating factors.
- ECG to establish precipitating factors.

The aim of treatment is to correct dehydration and electrolyte imbalance, hyperglycaemia, and the blood acidity. This is achieved by rapid replacement of fluid, electrolytes, and insulin, usually given intravenously.

The key to successful management of DKA is continued monitoring of glucose levels, electrolytes, urinary and plasma ketones, and regular reassessment in the first 12–24h. Intravenous insulin infusion should be on a sliding scale (see Table 8.1).

Table 8.1 Example of a sliding scale intravenous insulin infusion

Blood glucose level (mmol/l)	Short-acting insulin infusion rate (units/h)
0–3.9	0.5
4.0–8.0	1
8.1–12	2
12.1–16	3
16.1+	4

Source Page and Hall (1999).

Further information

Page S, Hall G. (1999) *Diabetes emergency and hospital management*. BMJ Publishing, London.

Hyperosmolar non-ketotic coma

Hyperosmolar non-ketotic coma is less common than DKA and usually occurs in the older age group, predominantly in patients who are >60 years of age. It is a complication of Type 2 diabetes and may be the initial presentation in approximately 30% of cases.

Physiology

HONK occurs as a result of severe hyperglycaemia, marked dehydration, and electrolyte loss. Osmotic diuresis is a key clinical feature, but this tends to be more insidious in onset and develop more slowly. The key difference to DKA is the absence of ketones.

Precipitating causes

- Infection or underlying illness, such as myocardial infarction, CVA.
- Thiazide or loop diuretics.
- Beta blockers.
- Corticosteroids.

Clinical features

- Polyuria, polydipsia.
- Lethargy weakness general malaise.
- Confusion and disorientation.
- Hypotension.
- Disturbed level of consciousness.

Treatment

The principles of treatment for HONK are similar to DKA – rehydration with isotonic saline to restore bp. Rehydration tends to be carried out with more caution, as the patients in this age group tend to be more elderly and often have co-existing cardiovascular disease. An insulin infusion is often given to correct hyperglycaemia. Anti-coagulation therapy is often commenced as the risk of thrombosis is greater with HONK than DKA. For the differences between HONK and DKA see Table 8.2.

Following initial treatment, insulin may be necessary for a short period until the patient is fully recovered. This is often determined by the precipitating factor and the patient's recovery from this. It is unusual for the patient to need long-term insulin.

Table 8.2 Differences between DKA & HONK

Factor	DKA	HONK
Age	Any	Usually >60 years
Presentation	Hours or days	Days or weeks
Mortality	5% overall	50%
Glucose	High	Very high
Osmolarity	High	Very high
Serum sodium	Normal or low	Normal or high
Bicarbonate	< 15	Normal or slightly low
Ketonuria	++++	None
Treatment	IV insulin/ insulin	Insulin initially then diet and often oral hypoglycaemic agents

Reproduced from Page S and Hall G (1999), *Diabetes Emergency and Hospital Management*, with permission from Wiley Blackwell.

Further information

Page S, Hall G. (1999) *Diabetes Emergency and Hospital Management.* BMJ Publishing, London.

Steroid-induced diabetes

Pharmacological doses of corticosteroids may precipitate the development of diabetes. Corticosteroids increase insulin resistance and, therefore, result in hyperglycaemia. Those most at risk of developing steroid-induced diabetes include those with a previous history of gestational diabetes or previous history of glucose intolerance.

Effects of steroids on established diabetes

Corticosteroids typically cause a small rise in fasting BG levels and a marked increased in post-prandial BG levels. The hyperglycaemic effects are usually temporary and related to the dose of steroids; typically, this resolves when the steroids are stopped.

Treatment

As the effect on BG levels can be dramatic changes in diabetes medication may be required, increasing sulphonyureas may be necessary or, in some cases, insulin may be needed. This will need to be reviewed as steroid doses are reduced and stopped.

Other endocrine disorders

People with diabetes have a greater risk of developing other endocrine disorders; the development of other endocrine disorders may influence BG control, routine screening for thyroid disorders is typically carried out annually.

Thyroid disorders

Thyrotoxicosis

Caused by excessive thyroid hormone, there are numerous causes of thyrotoxicosis.

Signs and symptoms

- Hyperactivity.
- Heat intolerance, sweating, warm skin.
- Palpitations.
- Weight loss.
- Pruritus.
- Thirst and polyuria.
- Hair loss.
- Fatigue, weakness.

Myoedema

Caused by insufficient levels of thyroid hormone.

Signs ands symptoms

- Fatigue, lethargy.
- Weight gain, despite decreasing appetite.
- Dry skin, hair loss.
- Deep hoarse voice.

There is an increased risk of thyroid disorders in diabetes. Thyrotoxicosis is associated to Type 1 diabetes and if thyroxine levels are elevated fluctuations in BG levels may occur.

Acromegaly

Caused by excessive production of growth hormone.

Signs and symptoms

- Lethargy.
- Headaches.
- Joint pains.
- Increased sweating.
- Change in ring or shoe size.
- Enlarged hands feet.
- Deep voice.
- Coarse facial features.

Effects on BG levels

Acromegaly increases insulin resistance and glucose intolerance, and therefore BG levels may rise at the onset.

Long-term complications

Risk factors for development: duration of diabetes

The United Kingdom Prospective Diabetes Study (UKPDS) of people with Type 2 diabetes and the Diabetes Control and Complications Trial (DCCT) of those with Type 1 have demonstrated a correlation between the development of long-term complications of diabetes and the length of time the person has the condition (see Table 9.1). This may be due to a combination of exposure to elevated circulating BG levels (DCCT and UKPDS), and the interaction between genetic and environmental factors. The major environmental risk factors are outlined under the following headings:

- Hypertension.
- Smoking.
- Higher body mass index.
- High waist circumference.
- Lipid disorders.

Table 9.1 Frequently seen long-term complications of diabetes

Area effected	Causing
Microvascular	Renal disease
	Eye disease
	Foot problems
Macrovascular	Stroke (CVA)
	Myocardial infarctions (MI)
	Foot problems
Nerve damage	Erectile dysfunction (ED)
	Foot problems
Other	Depression

Further information

Diabetes Control and Complications Trial Research Group (DCCT) (1996). The absence of a glycemic threshold for the development of long-term complications: the perspective of the Diabetes Control and Complications Trial. *Diabetes* **45**, 1289–98.

United Kingdom Prospective Diabetes Study (UKPDS) Group (1993). Intensive blood-glucose control with sulphonylureas or insulin compared with conventional treatment and risk of complications in patients with Type 2 diabetes. (UKPDS 33). *Lancet* **352**, 837–53.

Risk factors for development: metabolic control

Both the UKPDS and DCCT have provided evidence for the long-held view that metabolic control is implicated in the development of long-term complications in people with diabetes. Fioretto et al. (1998) reported that patients who have received pancreatic transplants, before they had developed end-stage renal failure, show a lessening or reversal of their renal lesions, which they argue must be as a result of their improved metabolic control following transplantation.

To reduce risk factors it is important to tread a difficult path between tight glycaemic control and the risk of episodes of frequent hypoglycaemia.

The National Institute for Clinical Excellence (NICE) (2008) guidelines suggest haemoglobin A1c (HbA1c) levels of 6.5% for people with diabetes.

Self-monitoring of BG levels both before (pre-prandial) and after (post-prandial) meals and adjustment of treatment in accordance with the results is an important factor in achieving acceptable levels of glycaemic control. NICE (2008) suggest people with Type 2 diabetes should aim to keep their pre-prandial glucose levels below 7.0mmol/l and post-prandial below 8.5mmol/l. (NICE, 2008)

For people with Type 2 diabetes it is important to check their local guidelines as recommendations vary; however, pre-prandial glucose levels of between 5 and 7mmol/l, and post-prandial results below 10mmol/l are generally appropriate.

For people with Type 1 diabetes, NICE (2004) guidelines suggest:
• Pre-prandial levels between 4 and 7mmol/l
• Post-prandial levels below 9mmol/l.

Further information

Fioretto P, Steffes MW, Goetz FC, Sutherland DER, Mauer M. (1998) Pancreatic transplantation and diabetic control. *N Engl J Med* **339**, 115–17.

National Institute for Clinical Excellence (NICE) (2004) *Type 1 diabetes: diagnosis and management of Type 1 diabetes in children, young people and adults. (CG 15).* National Collaborating Centre for Women's and Children's Health and the National Collaborating Centre for Chronic Conditions, London. Available at: 🖳 http://www.nice.org.uk/nicemedia/pdf/CG015NICEguideline.pdf (accessed 4 December 2008).

National Institute for Clinical Excellence (NICE) (2008) *Clinical guideline (CG66) for Type 2 diabetes.* National Collaborating Centre for Chronic Conditions, London. Available at: 🖳 http://www.nice.org.uk/nicemedia/pdf/CG66NICEGuideline.pdf (accessed 4 December 2008).

Risk factors for development: blood pressure and lipid control

Cardiovascular disease (CVD) is the major cause of morbidity and mortality in people with diabetes, and coronary heart disease is the most common cause of death among people with Type 2 diabetes. Elevated blood pressure (bp) and an abnormal lipid profile are both indicators of raised risk for arterial complications of diabetes. See 📖 Blood test results: lipid profiles, p. 128.

Microalbuminuria is present in about 80% of people with Type 1 diabetes before the onset of hypertension (Oster et al 1990). UKPDS showed 38% of newly-diagnosed patients with Type 2 diabetes had hypertension defined as repeated bp readings >160/90mmHg (150/85mmHg for those on antihypertensive medication). In the years following diagnosis the incidence of hypertension in those with Type 2 diabetes is greater than in an age-matched general population. This is an early indicator of renal disease (see 📖 Nephropathy, p. 208).

The bp control study (FACET 1997), which treated people with Type 2 diabetes to reduce their bp to an average of 144/82mmHg, showed significant reductions in risk:
- 24% for any diabetes relayed end-point.
- 32% for diabetes-related deaths.
- 44% for stroke.
- 37% for microvascular disease.
- 56% for heart failure.
- 34% for retinopathy progression.
- 47% for deterioration of vision.
(Oster et al 1990)

NICE guidelines CG15 and CG66 (2004a) suggest different bp and lipid targets for those with Type 1 diabetes and those with Type 2 diabetes see Tables 9.2 and 9.3).

Lipid control

Diabetes UK suggests targets should be:
- Total cholesterol level below 4.0mmol/l.
- LDL levels less than 2.0mmol/l.
- HDL levels 1.0mmol/l or above in men and 1.2mmol/l or above in women.
- Triglyceride levels 1.7mmol/l or less.

In order to rule secondary causes assess:
- Alcohol consumption and liver function to check it is not secondary to liver disease.
- Thyroid function to exclude hyperthyroidism.
- Serum creatinine and urine protein to exclude renal disease.

Management of those with abnormal lipid profiles

- Optimize glycaemic control (HbA1c below 6.5%).
- Advise on diet and physical activity.
- Weight loss advice for those who are overweight or obese.
- If the lipid profile shows a high risk of CVD, consider a statin.

Table 9.2 NICE guidance regarding elevated bp levels for people with Type 1 diabetes (NICE, 2008) and Type 1 diabetes (NICE, 2004a)

Type 2 diabetes	Type 1 diabetes
Repeat bp measurements within	Intervention is required if bp
1month if bp is higher than 150/90mmHg	Above 135/85mmHg
2months if bp is higher than 140/80mmHg	
2months if bp is higher than 130/80mmHg, and there is kidney, eye or cerebrovascular damage.	
Offer lifestyle advice (diet and exercise) at the same time.	Above 130/85mmHg for those with abnormal albumin excretion rates or another symptom of metabolic syndrome

Table 9.3 NICE guidance regarding lipid management

Type 2 Diabetes (2008)	Type 1 Diabetes (2004)
Before starting lipid-modifying therapy carry out a full lipid profile: High-density lipoprotein [HDL] Cholesterol Triglyceride	Recommend intervention in the reduction of risk factors for those who are over 35 years with: A family history of CVD High risk ethnic groups Those with hypertension Abnormal blood lipids
All people with Type 2 diabetes are considered to be at high cardiovascular risk unless they are: Not overweight Normotensive Without microalbuminurea A non-smoker No high risk lipid profile No personal or family history of CVD	

Further information

Diabetes UK. Treatment & your health. 🖥 www.diabetes.org.uk/Guide-to-diabetes/Treatment__ your_health (accessed 15 April 2009).

Appropriate Blood Pressure Control in Diabetes (ABCD) study (1997). Fosinopril versus Amlodipine Cardiovascular Events Randomised Trial (FACET). *Circulation* **96** (S1), 1.764i.

NICE (2004a) *Clinical guideline (CG15) for Type 1 diabetes adults*, Quick Reference Guide. Available at: 🖥 www.nice.org.uk/guidance/index.jsp?action=download&o=29391 (accessed 14 April 2008).

NICE (2004b) *Clinical Guideline G Management of Type 2 diabetes*. Available at: 🖥 www.nice.org. uk/nicemedia/pdf/NICE_INHERITEG_guidelines (accessed 14 April 2008).

NICE (2008) *Type 2 diabetes: the management of Type 2 diabetes (update)*. Available at: 🖥 www. nice.org.uk/CG66 (accessed 17 June 2009).

Oster JR, Masterson BJ, Eptein M. (1990) Diabetes mellitus and hypertension. *Cardiovasc Risk Factors* **1**, 25.

Risk factors for development: weight and abdominal adiposity

Being overweight increases insulin resistance and this has implications for everyone. Carrying excess weight around the waist (abdominal adiposity) is especially problematic for the utilization of insulin, either injected or endogenous, and especially for those of South Asian decent.

South Asians have a higher propensity to develop Type 2 diabetes and have higher risks for cardiovascular disease. Weight alone is not a good indicator of their risk factor and abdominal adiposity should be measured instead (see 📖 Chapter 7, pp. 119–160; 📖 Risk factors for development: metabolic control, p. 181).

Jung (1977) has suggested the health benefits of 10% weight loss are:
- 50% reduction in the risk of developing diabetes.
- Fall in bp of 10mmHg systolic and fall of 20mmHg diastolic.
- 30–50% fall in fasting BG.
- 15% decrease in HbA1c.
- 10% decrease in total cholesterol.
- 15% decrease in LDL cholesterol.
- 30% decrease in triglycerides.
- 8% increase in HDL cholesterol.

Further information
Jung RT. (1977) Obesity as a disease. *Br Med Bull* **53**, 307–21.

Risk factors for development: smoking

People with diabetes who smoke double their risk factors for developing cardiovascular disease.

Smoking also increases the risks of:
- Neuropathy.
- Nephropathy.
- Retinopathy.
- Stroke.
- Increased LDL.
- Lower HDL.
- Increase atherosclerosis.
- Prolongs time it takes to heal foot and leg ulcers.
- Increased adrenalin, which elevates bp.
- Nicotine may be implicated in insulin resistance.

See also 📖 Chapter 12, pp. 265–290.

Risk factors for development: genetics

MODY 2 (HNF4α)

Although extremely rare, comprising about 0.0001% of all Type 2 and about 5% of MODY people with this profile, it carries the risk of severe hyperglycaemia and, therefore, a high frequency of microvascular complications

MODY 2 (glucokinase)

- Less than 0.2% of Type 2.
- 10% of MODY cases.
- Only mild hyperglycaemia, therefore, low genetic risk for long-term complications.

MODY 3 (HNF1α)

- About 1–2% of people with Type 2.
- About 70% of MODY.
- Can give severe hyperglycaemia and, therefore, a high frequency of microvascular complications.

Being of either South Asian or Afro-Caribbean genetic origin will increase the risk of developing the microvascular complications of diabetes.

UKPDS has shown the increased risk of developing coronary heart disease (CHD) for people with Type 2 diabetes if they have an increased LDL-cholesterol and a decreased HDL-cholesterol, hypertension, hyperglycaemia, and are smokers. One suggested reason for this is that individuals within this group inherit a genetic predisposition to insulin resistance.

Some people with Type 1 diabetes may have a genetic predisposition to early renal disease associated with diabetic nephropathy, hypertension, and microalbuminurea (see 📖 Urine test results, p. 134).

It has been suggested that there may be a genetic link between hyper-insulinaemia, hypertension, and insulin resistance in people with Type 2 diabetes (see 📖 Chapter 2, p. 27).

Vascular complications

Both haemodynamic and biochemical changes (Boxes 9.1 and 9.2) in the blood supply are caused by hyperglycaemia, and result in impaired blood flow throughout large blood vessels (the macrovascular complications) and small blood vessels (the microvascular complications; Box 9.3).

Macrovascular complications

People with diabetes are at greater risk of macrovascular complications affecting the large blood vessels than those who do not have diabetes.

Macrovascular disease comprises:
- Coronary heart disease.
- Cerebrovascular disease.
- Peripheral vascular disease.

These comprise the cause of death in about 75% of patients with Type 2 diabetes and about 35% of deaths of those who have Type 1 diabetes.

The prevalence, incidence, and outcomes of these complications are mitigated by the following factors:
- Age.
- Sex.
- Ethnic genetic origin.

Although, histologically, the atheroma is the same throughout the whole population in those who have diabetes it:
- Is more diffuse.
- Progresses more quickly.
- Occurs at an earlier age.
- Affects both sexes equally (women with diabetes loose their pre-menopausal protection).

Compared with those with Type 2 diabetes, people with Type 1 diabetes have:
- ½ the rate of coronary heart disease.
- ⅓ the rate of cerebrovascular disease.
- ⅔ the rate of peripheral vascular disease.

Just as in the population at large, smoking and family history also comprise risk factors for atherosclerosis. People who have diabetes also have other common risk factors.

Glycaemic control
- In people with Type 1 diabetes, poor glycaemic control is related to the amount of atherosclerosis present.
- UKPDS suggests that is also true for those with Type 2 diabetes.

Hypertension is common in both types of diabetes. UKPDS suggests bp control is more important for those with Type 2 diabetes than glycaemic control.

Hyperlipidaemia is common in those with Type 2 diabetes where it causes a reduction in HDL cholesterol, elevated triglycerides, and VDL and an increase in small dense atherogenic LDL-cholesterol (see 📖 Cholesterol, p. 130).

Obesity is common in those with Type 2 diabetes and poses a more significant risk with abdominal adiposity.

Insulin resistance: elevated levels of circulating insulin increase the risk of atherosclerosis.

Box 9.1 Haemodynamic changes in hyperglycaemia

Causes of impaired microvascular flow:
- Increased tendency of circulating blood to coagulate.
- Increased viscosity.
- Platelet hypersensitivity.
- Microvascular sclerosis.
- Impaired flow causes: raised capillary pressure

Box 9.2 Biochemical changes in hyperglycaemia leading to tissue damage

- Intercellular glucose levels raised.
- Aldose reductase (enzyme in carbohydrate metabolism) increased.
- Intracellular sorbitol (a sugar alcohol) raised.
- Reduced intercellular myoinositol (a glucose isomer).
- Activation of protein kinase C (implicated in vasoconstriction).
- Increased glycation of proteins.
- Formation of advanced glycation end product (implicated in circulatory degeneration).

Box 9.3 Microvascular complications

Microvascular complications affect the small blood vessels and are causative in:
- Retinopathy.
- Nephropathy.
- Neuropathy.

Those with Type 1 diabetes are at a greater risk of developing these long-term complications than those with Type 2.

Primary risk factors are:
- Hyperglycaemia.
- Hypertension.
- Dislipidaemia.

Further information

Aronson D, Rayfield E (2002). How hyperglycaemia promotes atherosclerosis; molecular mechanism. *Cardiovasc Diabetol* **1**, 1. Available at: ☐ http://www.cardiab.com/content/1/1/1 (accessed on 4 December 2008).

Adeghate E, Saadi H, Adem A, Obineche E (2006). Diabetes mellitus and its complications: molecular mechanisms, epidemiology, and clinical medicine. *Annl NY Acad Sci* **1084**, 481–9.

Diabetic foot assessments

Introduction

The rationale for annual diabetic foot assessments is to identify patients who have risk factors for ulceration or amputation, and to provide appropriate foot-care and education. This approach has been shown to be successful in reducing severe foot complications. A foot assessment should consist of a full medical history, comprehensive foot examination, including neurological, vascular, joint and soft tissue assessments. All findings should be recorded in a clear, concise, and structured manner, with a recorded outcome. Remember, physically examining patients' feet gives a clear message that they are important.

History-taking

Taking a full medical and drug history alerts clinicians to the possibility of existing pathologies that affect the foot before any physical examination takes place. For example, macro- or microvascular diseases, e.g. hypertension, retinopathy, etc., may be suggestive of peripheral arterial disease.

Clinical observations

First observe the patient walking into the treatment room, noting any abnormalities of gait, e.g. shuffling, limping, high stepping gait, etc. Simple observations like this can easily go unnoticed. Always try to look for the obvious and compare with the contralateral side. Note the general skin condition, hair growth, nail pathologies, callus, dryness, fungal skin infections, discolouration, localized swelling, deformity, or evidence of previous ulceration or surgery. Inspect both feet systematically from toe to heel, not forgetting between the toes and the backs of the heels.

Examination

Always explain clearly what you are doing and why, before performing tests or examination. When finished ensure you share your findings with the patient. This reinforces patient education, empowerment, and self-care. Note whether the patient can see and reach their foot easily, as a reduced ability to do either of these increases the risk of complications considerably (see Table 9.4 for an assessment chart).

Skin fissures (splits) are common, especially on the heels. They can deteriorate rapidly to ulceration and necrosis in patients with neuro-ischaemia.

Plantar callus is common in the neuropathic foot and a high risk factor for ulceration, occurring over the metatarsal heads and toes. It is diffuse and thick. In contrast the neuro-ischaemic foot is typically thin, dry, glassy, and very hard. The presence of bloodstained callus is highly predictive of ulceration being present in up to 80% of cases following callus removal.

Nails: thickened nails are often distorted and discoloured, but not friable, affecting one or several toenails. They are caused by either a single major or repeated trauma. They can lead to ulceration of the nail bed, which may extend to bone, especially in patients with ischaemia. This requires referral to a podiatrist for treatment.

Fungal infections

Common skin sites are between the toes, presenting as wet or dry fissures, and under the medial arch, presenting as vesicular eruptions. Nail infections are characterized by thickened, discoloured, and friable nail plates. Although *Tinea pedis* does not primarily cause foot ulceration, secondary bacterial infection may lead to deep web-space ulceration, and thus *Tinea* should always be treated (skin, not nails) with an anti-fungal preparation, such as terbinafine. **NB.** Anti-fungal dusting powders are ineffective as a treatment for skin, but may be used preventatively in shoes and socks.

Foot deformity and joint mobility

These result from altered foot mechanics, poorly fitting footwear, neuropathy, and surgery. Deformities are significant when they are unable to be accommodated in a high street shoe. Ankle equinus, shortening of the Achilles tendon, is commonly associated with neuropathy and may contribute to forefoot ulceration.

Footwear

Ask patients to describe what shoes they wear daily. A suitable shoe should be laced or strapped, have adequate length and toe box depth, and an appropriate shape, i.e. rounded. Don't forget to look inside the shoes for rucked linings or foreign objects!

Key foot ulcer risk factors

Intrinsic ulcer risk factors

- Peripheral neuropathy.
- Peripheral arterial disease.
- Previous ulcer/amputation.
- Callus (neuropathy).
- Limited joint mobility.
- Deformity.
- Dry skin/fissures.
- Poor glycaemic control.

Extrinsic ulcer risk factors

- Infection (bacterial/fungal).
- High plantar pressures/trauma.
- Alcohol.
- Poor healthcare education, attitudes, or beliefs.
- Smoking.
- Poor podiatry provision.
- Inadequate footwear.

Table 9.4 Assessment outcomes

Assessment	Outcome	Score
Neuropathy evident	Yes (1)/No (0)	
Pulses absent(both in either foot)	Yes (1)/No (0)	
Callus with neuropathy	Yes (1)/No (0)	
Previous ulcer/amputation	Yes (2)/No (0)	
Deformity	Yes (1)/No (0)	
Inability to reach or see feet – a score for each	Yes (0–5)/No (0)	
Intermittent claudication/rest pain	Yes (1)/No (0)	

Ulcer risk score = 0–0.5 low risk, 1–1.5 medium risk, ≥2 high risk.

Reproduced with permission from Baker et al. (2005)

Further information

Baker N, et al. (2005) *Diabet Foot J* **8**. Information on foot screening and assessment is available throughout this volume of the journal.

Podiatry provision: foot-care protection services

Introduction

Podiatry services within the NHS are placed within the community and are accessible to all who have a foot problem that requires specialist help. However, priority is given to the elderly, children, the disabled, or those with a serious medical condition. Patients can access the service directly without referral, or can be referred by medical and non-medical staff. Not surprisingly, the demands on the service provision are high and, thus, in many areas are restricted to those with a medical need. Clearly, this applies to people with diabetes, but only if they are at risk for foot ulceration. Annual reviews of people with diabetes should include a foot examination identifying those with active foot ulcers, peripheral obstructive arterial disease (POAD), or ulcer risk. NICE Clinical Guideline 10 lays out a clear pathway for the prevention and management of such patients based on best current evidence.

Why podiatry is important

Podiatrists are trained to assess, diagnose, and treat foot conditions. Perhaps the two most important skills are debridement of callus (dead and devitalized tissue), and management of extrinsic and intrinsic pathomechanics. The presence of callus increases the risk of ulceration by up to 77 times in the neuropathic foot. Podiatrists are highly skilled at removing and preventing it. Meticulous nail care, especially in those with POAD and renal failure, is imperative in the fight against gangrene.

Recommended foot-care pathway

A dedicated diabetic foot-care protection team, ideally, should be available in every district. This should aim to provide an integrated diabetic foot-care between primary and secondary care for patients with current or potential foot problems. The pathway consists of 3 levels – screening, intermediate care for those with moderate or high risk, and specialist foot clinics for ulcerated, Charcot, infected, or critical ischaemia (see Fig 9.1).

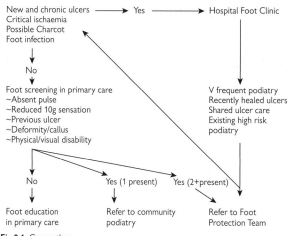

New and chronic ulcers ——→ Yes ——————→ Hospital Foot Clinic
Critical ischaemia
Possible Charcot
Foot infection

No

Foot screening in primary care
~Absent pulse
~Reduced 10g sensation
~Previous ulcer
~Deformity/callus
~Physical/visual disability

V frequent podiatry
Recently healed ulcers
Shared ulcer care
Existing high risk
podiatry

No   Yes (1 present)   Yes (2+present)

Foot education   Refer to community   Refer to Foot
in primary care   podiatry   Protection Team

Fig 9.1 Care pathway

NB. It is important to find out and use your local care pathways.

Foot risk classification

- **Low risk:** at least one pulse per foot, and able to feel 10g monofilament and/or vibration with no foot deformity or physical/visual impairment. An exception to otherwise low risk is those presenting with active bacterial or fungal skin infections. These should be treated as short term immediate high risk patients until the infection has been cleared.
- **Moderate risk:** unable to detect both pulses in a foot, or unable to feel 10g monofilament and/or vibration. No foot deformity, able to see or reach foot. No callus and no previous ulceration.
- **High risk:** previous ulcer or amputation and/or absent pulse and unable to feel 10g monofilament/vibration, plus one or more of the following:
  - callus, fixed deformity, partial/total blindness, unable to reach feet;
  - renal failure.
- **Extreme risk:** ulceration, patients with active ulceration, gangrene.

See Box 9.4 for management routes.

Box 9.4 Management of foot conditions by risk level

Low risk
- General foot-care advice + annual diabetes review.
- Assessed for routine podiatry needs.

Moderate risk
- Targeted/enhanced foot-care advice. Inspect 3–6-monthly.
- Footwear inspection and advice.
- Review vascular status regularly (6 months).

High risk
- Arrange frequent review (1–3-monthly) from specialized podiatry/ foot care team.
- At each regular diabetes review, evaluate the provision of:
  - intensified foot care education;
  - specialist footwear and insoles;
  - frequent (according to need) skin and nail care.
- Review education/footwear/vascular status as for the at risk foot
- Ensure special arrangements for those people with disabilities or immobility.

Extreme risk
- Urgently arrange foot ulcer care from a team with specialist expertise.
- Expect that team to ensure, as a minimum:
  - investigation and treatment of vascular insufficiency;
  - local wound management, appropriate dressings, and debridement as indicated;
  - systemic antibiotic therapy for cellulitis or bone infection;
  - effective means of distributing foot pressures, including specialist footwear, casts.
- Optimizing BG control.

Foot care emergency
- New ulceration, un-resolving cellulitis (3–4days), discolouration, acute Charcot, acute ischaemia.
- Refer to specialized podiatry/foot care team within 24h where possible or follow your local care pathway guidance.

Peripheral vascular complications: overview and presentation

Peripheral obstructive arterial disease (POAD) can be defined as lower extremity atherosclerosis. Arterial assessment should be grounded in a clear knowledge of anatomy and pathophysiology, together with the ability to take a comprehensive patient history

POAD reportedly occurs 20 times more often in people with diabetes compared with the general population. It is reported that POAD is the single most likely cause of lower extremity amputations in people with diabetes and, importantly, is more rapid in its progression occurring at younger age compared with the general population. However, ischaemia in patients with diabetes often co-exists with neuropathy, affecting up to 45% of foot ulcer patients.

Disease pattern

The distribution of arterial occlusive lesions varies from aorto-iliac disease to multi-segmental diffuse lesions extending to the ankle and foot. The tibio-peroneal trunk and crural vessels are most aggressively affected. Foot vessels are often spared, but due to 2–3 segmental level disease they are frequently not evident. Aneurysms of the aorta, iliac, and popliteal vessels are not uncommon. Arterial medial wall calcification is also very common, especially in patients with neuropathy and renal failure.

Presentation

The skin generally looks impoverished and fragile, appearing:
- Wrinkled.
- Dry, cool.
- There is little hair growth.
- Atrophy of the underlying dermal tissue.

The colour of the skin may vary from pale to dusky/deep red to mauve.

In pigmented skin colour change is less obvious, but generally appears darker and wrinkled.

The foot and leg may be oedematous with toes that look like 'beef chipolata'! The toenails are generally dystrophic (altered growth due to pathology or defective nutrition), being very thin or yellowed, and thick. They may be quite brittle, slow growing, and difficult to cut. If callus is present it is usually thin and hard, and not diffuse, generally occurring on the margins of the foot.

If an ulcer is present it is usually 'punched out' with a sloughy base occurring on the toes, foot borders, or dorsum. These lesions are painful, although this may be dulled due to co-existent neuropathy.

Peripheral vascular complications: diagnosis and treatment

Clinical tests and symptoms

Palpation of dorsalis pedis and posterior tibial pulses may be weak or absent. Remember that a palpable pulse does not always equate with good perfusion. In the absence of foot pulses, always examine for popliteal and femoral pulses. This gives an indication of disease distribution and is essential information for angiography referral. If a hand-held Doppler is used the audible signals are typically low pitched and monophasic in character.

Ankle systolic pressures can also be obtained using a hand-held Doppler and standard arm syphgmanometer. The normal ankle systolic pressure should be equal or up to 30mmHg greater than the brachial. Falsely elevated pressures due to medial wall calcification are common (see Table 9.5).

Elevation and dependency tests are useful here watching for pallor on elevation and 'sunset red' on dependency. The pole test is a modification of this, measuring the height at which the Doppler signal disappears on elevation with the patient supine. The lower the signal loss or pallor the greater the disease.

Intermittent claudication or rest pain may be present, but it is important to distinguish between ischaemic and neuropathic pain, or intermittent claudication and spinal stenosis.

Table 9.5 Ankle Pressure Index

Ankle Pressure Index	Interpretation of results
≥1–3	Test is meaningless – calcified vessels
0.8–1.2	No significant arterial disease evident
0.5–0.79	Suggestive of significant arterial disease
≤0.5	Suggestive of critical limb ischaemia

In summary it is very important not to arrive at a clinical diagnosis of POAD based purely upon one clinical test or observation, such as absent foot pulses or symptoms of rest pain (see Table 9.6).

Table 9.6 Clinical symptoms of POAD

Pain	Intermittent claudication	Rest pain	Neuropathic pain
Site	Foot/calf/thigh/buttock	Foot/lower leg	Foot/shin
Type	Cramp-like	Unremitting gnawing ache	Burning, shooting, stabbing, electric shocks, lacinating,
Onset	On exercise	At rest or on elevation	More noticeable at night
Relief	Rest	Lowering leg	Exercise
Other features	Weak/absent pulses ABPI <0.7	Absent pulses ABPI <0.5	Good pulses, warm healthy skin

Chronic critical limb ischaemia

Defined by either of the following two criteria:

- Persistently recurring ischaemic rest pain requiring analgesia for more than 2 weeks, with an ankle systolic pressure of ≥50mmHg and or a toe pressure of ≥30mmHg.
- Ulceration or gangrene of the foot or toes with an ankle systolic pressure of ≥50mmHg and or a toe pressure of ≥30mmHg.

Table 9.7

Observation	Suggested action
No clinical evidence of POAD	Annual review
Intermittent claudication (no ulcer/gangrene)	Encourage exercise, monitor CHD risk factors (bp, lipids, diet, exercise, smoking, etc.)
Evidence of POAD + ulceration/gangrene	Refer to specialist foot or vascular surgery clinic, check CHD management,
Non-healing neuro-ischaemic ulcer	Refer to specialist foot clinic
Rest pain	Refer for further investigation/opinion

Neuropathy: presentation, diagnosis, and treatment

Diabetic peripheral neuropathy can be defined as: 'the presence of symptoms and/or signs of peripheral nerve dysfunction in people with diabetes after other causes have been excluded' (Boulton et al, 1998).

Symmetrical peripheral distal polyneuropathy is common, affecting approximately 50% of people with Type 2 diabetes. Furthermore, up to 15% of people with diabetic neuropathy are likely to develop an ulcer in their lifetime.

Presentation

It is therefore clear from the evidence above that only a relatively small proportion of patients with peripheral neuropathy develop foot ulceration. Thus, annual foot screening should be directed at identifying those with ulcer risk due to neuropathy not neuropathy *per se*.

Peripheral neuropathy

Sensory loss is characterized as the absence or reduced ability to detect light, touch, pain, vibration, hot or cold. Frequently, patients describe pins and needles sensations, that their feet feel like cotton wool or that the feet feel cold even when warm to the touch. However, the most important characteristic is the inability to feel protective pain sensation manifesting as unnoticed injuries. **Autonomic** loss is generally subclinical, but the foot presents with dry, pink, warm skin, strong foot pulses, dilated dorsal veins, and some degree of oedema. Orthostatic hypotension may be identifiable.

Motor loss presents as feet that, on weight-bearing, have a high arch, claw toes, and a prominence of the metatarsal heads. Alterations in gait can be observed, e.g. unsteadiness, uncontrolled foot loading. In these situations there is usually accompanying proprioceptive loss, which is the loss of positional sense.

Symptomatic neuropathy

Painful diabetic neuropathy that may be acute or chronic occurs in up to 10% of patients. This is described as burning, shooting, lancinating, or stabbing pains, which are generally worse at night. Other symptoms include depression, insomnia, tiredness, and the inability to concentrate on a task. Paradoxically, both painless and painful neuropathy can be present in patients. Always exclude other causes of neuropathy, e.g. alcoholism, vitamin B12 deficiency (pernicious anaemia; be aware that metformin can decrease vitamin B12 absorption), etc.

Allodynia is another form of painful neuropathy in which the skin becomes exquisitely tender to the touch.

Sensory tests

There are several commonly used screening tools used for determining neuropathic ulcer risk including:

- 10g monofilament.
- Cotton wool.
- 128Hz tuning fork Neurotips™.
- Hot/cold rods.
- Neurothesiometer™.

Not all the sensory testing equipment has a good evidence base for practice. Therefore, the recommended neuropathic ulcer risk screening tool(s) in everyday use are the 10g monofilament and/or 128Hz tuning fork (see Box 9.5). However, tools are only as good as the person using them and, therefore, results from sensory testing should be used in conjunction with other risk factors.

Box 9.5 Most commonly used clinical testing methods

- **Nylon monofilaments:** 10g (for light pressure).
- **Tuning fork:** 128Hz (for vibration).
- **Neuropen™:** combines 10g monofilament and Neurotip on a calibrated spring all incorporated in a pen-like device.
- **Neurothesiometer™:** measures vibration perception in volts.
- **Neurotip™:** may be used with or without Neuropen™ for sharp sensation or using both ends for distinguishing between sharp and blunt sensations. Hot and cold metal rods or water-filled test tubes (for temperature appreciation).
- **Tendon reflexes:** ankle and knee jerk.
- **Neuropathy symptom scores.**
- **Neuropathy disability scores.**

How to use a 10g nylon monofilament (NMF)

- Buckle a couple of times before testing.
- Pre-test on a sensitive area of patient's skin, e.g. inside of forearm.
- With eyes closed patient says YES every time they feel any contact.
- Place at 90° to the skin surface avoiding callused or scar tissue.
- The 3 'ones' (do not 'jab' with the monofilament):
  - apply over 1s;
  - hold for 1s;
  - release over 1s.
- Record responses, if in doubt retest questioned sites.
- If the patient says NO, whilst testing they are really saying YES!

The inability to detect 1 or more sites on each foot = neuropathy.

Vibration perception

Using a 128Hz tuning fork, press the tips of the limbs together and sharply pull away your fingers. Place the vibrating tuning fork on the apex of the great toe. Ask the patient to describe what they feel, record their ability to feel vibration. Repeat on the other foot. Remember to pre-test elsewhere, e.g. the elbow.

Neuropathy Disability Score

This simple assessment uses a scoring system in which the patient scores one point for each incorrect test and an extra point if the Achilles tendon reflexes are not determined with reinforcement. The maximum score for each foot is 5 points, and a score of ≥3 out of 10 suggests neuropathy and ulcer risk.

Table 9.8 Neuropathy Disability Score

Assessment		Right	Left	Score
Neurotip discrimination	Dorsum hallux proximal to nail			
Temperature discrimination	Dorsum hallux proximal to nail			
Reflexes	Achilles tendon	0/R/2	0/R/2	
128 Hz tuning fork	Tip of hallux			
Total Score				

Reproduced with permission from Baker et al (2005).

Further information

Baker N, et al. (2005) *Diabet Foot J* **8**. Information on foot screening and assessment is available throughout this volume of the journal.

Nephropathy

Nephropathy, previously called diabetic renal disease, affects people with Type 1 and Type 2 diabetes. It is present in at least 17% of patients and is a major cause of premature death for these patients. The onset of the condition is gradual and regular urine testing for protein (microalbuminurea) is required for detection. Nephropathy is usually associated with diabetic retinopathy or neuropathy and systemic hypertension.

Epidemiology

- People with Type 1 diabetes:
  - nephropathy will occur in up to 35% of people;
  - more common in men diagnosed Type 1 before 15 years of age;
  - of those with proteinuria, 2/3 will develop renal failure (particularly those within the ethnic groups outlined below);
  - in the UK neuropathy causes 15% of all deaths in patients under 50.
- People with Type 2 diabetes have racial differences:
  - up to 50% of people of an Asian background develop nephropathy;
  - up to 25% of Caucasians expected to develop nephropathy;
  - nephropathy develops more quickly after diagnosis in this group, but this may be due to later diagnosis for Type 2 than Type 1 (see 📖 Incidence and epidemiology, p. 28).

A diagnosis may be made if a patient who has no other renal disease, heart failure, or urinary tract infection has persistent or intermittent proteinuria.

Positive results for microalbumin tests give an early indication of the disease. The onset of microalbuminuria is usually 5–15 years following the onset of the disease in those with Type 1 diabetes, but may be present at diagnosis in those with Type 2. The UKPDS, based on 3867 patients, suggest that about 12% have microalbuminuria (although using a high threshold) and 1.9% have proteinuria at the time of diagnosis of diabetes.

Testing regimes may vary within local protocols, but the implementation group for the St. Vincent Declaration[1] recommend that all patients with a negative protein on conventional dip stick should be annually screened for microalbuminuria:
- **Men with a urinary albumin:** creatinine ratio >2.5mg/mmol.
- **Women with a urinary albumin:** creatinine ratio >3.5mg/mmol.
- **Anyone with a positive urine dip test:** urine albumin >20µg.
- All patients should have a 24h timed urine collection repeated 3 times.

Predisposing factors

Hyperglycaemia

The DCCT showed that people with Type 1 diabetes who improved their glycaemic control had a reduction in their levels of microalbuminurea. This was also indicated in the UKPDS for those with Type 2 diabetes.

Systemic hypertension

- 85% of those with Type 1 diabetes who have nephropathy are hypertensive.
- Increased intraglomerular pressure is associated with hypertension.

Genetic predisposition

There is evidence of a genetic predisposition to develop nephropathy.

Smoking

A link between smoking and nephropathy has been established.

Table 9.9 Reading results for patients with no other predispositions, e.g. urinary tract infection, heart disease, or other renal impairment.

Test	Procedure	Diagnosis threshold
Proteinuria	1. Dip stick	Urinary protein >0.5g/24h
	2. Timed urine collection either over night or over a 24h period	
Albuminuria	1. Timed urine collection either over night or over a 24h period	Urinary albumin excretion rate >3000mg/24h or >200µg/min
Microalbuminuria	1. A clean-catch midstream urine sample, preferably a morning specimen*	Urinary albumin excretion rate 30–300mg/day or 20–200µg/min
Estimated glomerula filtration rates eGFR	This is an estimation using serum creatinine, age, gender and weight to calculate creatinine clearance. Calculations may be done using 🖳 http://www.renal.org/eGFRcalc/GFR.pl	Early diabetes- increased GFR The decline in GFR varies substantially form patient to patient: 2–20ml/min per year

*****NB** False positive for microalbuminuria may be obtained if the patient has been exercising, has a urinary tract infection or the specimen was contaminated by menstruation or semen.

Retinopathy: diabetic eye disease

There are a number of conditions of the eye associated with diabetes:
- **Cataracts:** more common in people with diabetes.
- **Diabetic retinopathy:** a long-term microvascular complication of diabetes.

Diabetic retinopathy (DR)
- The leading cause of blindness in the working population of the UK.
- It is unusual for those with Type 1 diabetes to develop DR in the first 5 years.
- 90% of those with Type 1 diabetes have DR within 20 years of diagnosis.
- 40% of those with Type 2 diabetes show signs of DR at diagnosis.
- More common in ethnic minority populations than Caucasians.

DR describes the process of change in the normal vascular structure of the retina. The retina is comprised of cells called rods and cones, which are light sensitive and create visual images via the optic nerve. The macula and fovea occupy the central part of the retina, and are responsible for detailed and central vision.

Predisposing factors
- **Hyperglycaemia:** impairs retinal perfusion and causes endothelial cell malfunction, resulting in a thickened capillary basement membrane.
- **Hypertension:** for both the development and progression of DR.
- **Hyperlipidaemia.**
- **Duration of diabetes.**
- **Genetic predisposition.**

Stages of retinopathy

The earliest evidence of DR is **background retinopathy** (BR) which is symptomless and requires fundoscopy to be detected. However, if BR occurs near the macula, maculopathy, loss of vision may be experienced.

Intensification of glycaemic control may accelerate BR progression initially.

The next stage is called **pre-proliferative retinopathy** (PPR). Cotton wool spots, seen on fundoscopy as white areas, are caused by nerve damage due to poor blood supply from occluded vessels. Irregularly-shaped blood vessels, intraretinal microvascular abnormalities (IRMAs) appear within the retina to try to combat the growing ischaemia. PPR is an important predictor of impending visual loss, requiring urgent opthamological referral.

Proliferative retinopathy describes the stage when in response to the increasing ischemia new vessels are produced either on the disc (NVD) or elsewhere (NVE). These vessels are weak and prone to haemorrhage and bleeding into the vitreous occurs. If unchecked, the cycle of bleeding and the resultant scarring will lead to blindness, and contraction of the scar tissue may also cause the retina to become detached. About 60% of people with PR will become blind within 5 years if they do not receive corrective treatment.

Maculopathy. The 5% of the retina central to the eye is called the macula. Vascular leakages at any stage of retinopathy will lead to the deposit of exudates which form a ring in the macula referred to as circinate exudate. Maculopathy may be described as 'focal' when the leaking vessels are localized or 'diffuse' if they are generalized.

Laser oblation. The aim of this treatment is to seal the leaking vessels and oblate new vessels. This stops the ischaemic stimulation of growth factors, which result in the formation of new vessels.

See Box 9.6.

Box 9.6 Stages of diabetic retinopathy and treatment

Background retinopathy (BR) is characterized by:
- Microaneurysms, seen as dots on the retina via fundoscopy.
- Haemorrhages.
- Hard exudates, where proteins and lipids leak from the blood vessels (seen as white dots).

Treatment: no treatment available, but careful monitoring **recommended.**

Preproliferative retinopathy (PPR) is characterized by:
- Soft exudates (appearing as cotton wool spots) are as a result of infarcts in the nerve fibre layer of the eye.
- Intraretinal microvascular abnormalities (IRMA's).
- Venous abnormalities: beading, looping and duplication.

Proliferative retinopathy (PR) is characterized by:
- New vessels growing within the retina, into the vitreous and even across the iris (the later known as rubeosis iridis).
- New vessels on the disc (NVD).
- New vessels elsewhere (NVE).
- Vitreous haemorrhage.
- Retinal detachment.

Treatment: laser oblation successful in about 80% of cases. Retinal detachment will require microsurgery and laser photocoagulation.

Maculopathy is characterized by:
- Haemorrhage and hard exudates in the macular area.
- Drop in visual acuity (see 📖 Visual acuity and retinal screening, p. 144) due to macula oedema.
- Loss of central or detailed vision due to macula oedema.
- Loss of colour vision.
- Can occur in either or both eyes.

Treatment: circinate exudates may be treated with focal laser therapy, whereas diffuse conditions require a grid of laser successful in about 60% of cases if begun before visual acuity has dropped.

NB. Rapid acceleration of retinopathy can occur during pregnancy. It is important that's screening is carried out pre-conceptually where possibly and regularly during pregnancy. Laser treatment is suitable where indicated.

Further reading

Full colour plate illustrations of fundoscopy maybe found in many text books, for example:
Williams G, Pickup J. (2004) *Handbook of diabetes*, 3rd edn. Blackwell Publishing, Oxford.

Diabetic retinopathy prevention

The aim of care for people with DR is the prevention of loss of sight through either primary or secondary causes. This requires strategies to optimize glycaemic and bp control, and to provide effective retinal screening. (See Box 9.7 for symptoms of diabetic retinopathy.)

Glycaemic and blood pressure control

Targets for good control and the reduction of risk factors for DR for both Type 1 (DCCT) or Type 2 (UKPDS) diabetes are:
- HbA1c below 7%.
- bp less than 140/80mmHg.

A reduction of 1% in HBA1c in people with Type 2 diabetes is associated with a decreased risk of microvascular complications.

Groups of people, such as pregnant women who achieve rapid improvements in glycaemic control may suffer a worsening of their retinopathy. It is therefore important to carefully monitor such groups over the subsequent 2 years.

Strategies for improving control
- Making sure insulin regimens and/or oral therapies are appropriate.
- Titrate dose to BG results.
- Look at exercise regimes.
- Recap on dietary advice and actual patterns of eating.

Guidelines for retinal screening programmes may vary locally. NICE offer guidelines for screening those with Type 2 diabetes.

Box 9.7 Symptoms of retinopathy

- Blurred vision.
- Appearance of floaters in the field of vision.
- Red, black, or grey spots in the eyes.
- Red or black wavy lines or 'spiders webs' in the visual field.
- A curtain like effect in particular area of vision.
- Flashes in the eye.
- Inability to focus on close work.
- Rapid and painless deterioration of vision.

Note, not all retinopathy leads to symptoms.

Further information

The Diabetes Control and Complications Trial Research Group (DCCT) (1996) The absence of a glycaemic threshold for the development of long-term complications: the perspective of the Diabetes Control and Complications Trial. *Diabetes* **45**, 1289–98.

UK Prospective Diabetes Study (UKPDS) Group (1998) Intensive blood-glucose control with sulphonylureas or insulin compared with conventional treatment and risk of complications in patients with Type 2 diabetes (UKPDS 33). *Lancet* **352**, 837–53.

National Institute for Clinical Excellence (NICE) (2008) *Clinical Guideline (CG66) for Type 2 diabetes*. National Collaborating Centre for Chronic Conditions, London. Available at: ⊑ http://www.nice.org.uk/nicemedia/pdf/CG66NICEGuideline.pdf (accessed 4 December 2008).

Skin conditions

Vitiligo

A skin condition mainly associated with Type 1 diabetes. Resulting from the destruction of the cells, which produce skin pigmentation, and most commonly affecting the chest and abdomen. However, the patches of discoloured skin may also occur around the mouth, nostrils, and eyes.

Treatments include the application of topical steroids or micropigmentation (tattooing). A high factor sun block needs to be used in sunlight to prevent the unprotected skin areas from burning.

Scleroderma diabeticorum

This rare condition mainly affects those with Type 2 diabetes and causes the skin of the back of the neck and upper back to thicken. Good glycaemic control and the use of moisturizers to soften skin are indicated.

Digital sclerosis (also known as diabetic cheiroarthropathy)

Skin of the toes, fingers, and hands become thickened and waxy in appearance sometimes causing stiffness in the finger joints (demonstrated by the prayer sign inability to straighten fingers). Improved glycaemic control is indicated.

Necrobiosis lipoidica diabeticorum (NLD)

Thought to result in changes in the balance of collagen and fat within the layers of the dermis the skin appears thin, reddened, and is often itchy and painful. The borders between the lesions and the rest of the skin are well defined.

Skin problems linked to diabetes and insulin resistance

Acanthosis nigricans

Mainly affecting the skin folds of the armpits, breast, side and back of the neck, and groin. The skin becomes darker, thicker, and velvety in appearance.

Seen as an indicator of diabetes and often affecting those who are overweight, the condition is often improved by weight loss.

Skin problems linked to atherosclerosis

When the atherosclerosis affects the blood vessels which supply the skin, changes occur due to the:
- diminished oxygen supply causing:
  - hair loss
  - thinning and shinny skin (especially shins)
  - cold skin
  - thickened discoloured toe nails.
- diminished numbers of white blood cells, which can lead slow healing of the lower limbs and feet.

Diabetic dermopathy

Shiny red oval lesions, sometimes called shin spots, which may be hot or itchy. No treatment is necessary.

Eruptive xanthomatosis
This condition may occur with the combination of high BG and triglyceride levels. Usually occurring on the buttocks, face, back of the arms, and underside of the legs, these waxy yellow pea-sized bumps, surrounded within a red halo, are often itchy. Reduction of the raised glucose and triglyceride levels are indicated.

Chapter 10

Erectile dysfunction

Overview

Definition

Erectile dysfunction (ED) has been defined as:

> The persistent inability to attain and maintain an erection sufficient for performance.
>
> Although as ED is not perceived as a life threatening condition it is closely associated with important physical conditions and may affect psychological health. As such ED has a significant impact on the quality of life on the patient and their partners.
>
> (Feldman et al, 1994)

ED is a common complication of diabetes and, although common, is rarely mentioned and/or discussed by patients and healthcare professionals (HCP) alike. Studies indicate that between 30–60% of men with diabetes has this complication. (Sethia and Eardley, 2003).

ED can occur in men with both Type 1 and Type 2 diabetes and in relation to other complications. The pathophysiology of ED and diabetes is multifactorial, and the roles of neuropathy and arteriopathy are well recognized. Diabetes can cause autonomic neuropathy which may lead to ED (Eardly and Sethia, 2003).

ED is not a single incidence of erectile failure, but when failure is more than 75% of the time during attempted intercourse. ED is not the same as having low sexual desire, or having problems with ejaculation and orgasm.

Pharmaceutical advances over recent years, especially in the development of the PDE5s, together with a higher profile of this complication has raised awareness, but there is still reluctance amongst men with diabetes to disclose this problem. Research evidence identifies that it may take up to 5 years for men to admit to having ED. Nurses can help search and identify the problem, explain the treatment options, and refer or initiate treatments as required.

Physiology of an erection

For an erection to occur, the brain needs visual and/or sexual stimulation to activate the autonomic nervous system. When stimulation occurs, neurotransmitters are released via the parasympathetic nervous system. This results in dilatation of the penile artery leading to increased blood supply to the penis and into the corpora cavernosa. Venous return of blood from the penis becomes reduced and the erection develops.

Detumescence of the penis occurs via the sympathetic nervous system. Blood flow reduces into the corpora cavernosa and venous return from the penis increases so the penis becomes flaccid. See Fig. 10.1 for a diagram of male genital anatomy.

Symptoms of erectile dysfunction

Symptoms of ED can be described as being organic or psychological in origin (see Table 10.1). However, most organic causes of ED will also have a component of psychological ED. Men with ED will often describe feelings of anxiety or a fear of being unable to obtain or maintain an erection.

the question about erectile
ction

often be the best placed HCP to help identify ED in men with

ng the topic

onsultation it may help to talk in the third person, i.e. 'Men
mes get problems with their erections and this is something
able to help with, is this something you would like to discuss
/or take information about?' Once this topic is opened up it
ve permission for the individual to discuss the problem. It is
ng that this can often be denied initially, but returned to at
sultation. Evidence suggests that often it may be up to 5 years
fore an individual will disclose to a HCP that they have an issue
urse Education in Erectile Dysfunction (NEED), 2005]. Factors
to discussing ED should be considered prior to a consultation –
rs of persons present at the consultation and confidentiality
two examples. Other factors may have to be taken into con-
such as gender issues between a female nurse and a male
is may be overcome by observing the patient's body language
onsultation and, if necessary, asking if the patient would prefer
issues in relation to ED with a HCP of the same sex. In some
ups, a female nurse asking questions regarding sexual matters
cause of embarrassment and offence for some male patients.
be that some male patients have issues regarding discussion of
ith another male. The authors feel that the use of a male lan-
ort worker can be invaluable in some circumstances.

of ED, if discussed in a matter-of-fact way, with explanation as
nay be a complication of diabetes, can be reassuring to patients
artners, making them more willing to discuss the issues relating
) problem. Patients may sometimes not wish to discuss ED for
parrassment.

e patient disclose that he has ED, this can then be an opportu-
how this may affect his quality of life and/or relationships.

i may not be aware that diabetes can cause ED. Mentioning this
on during education in relation to diabetes is helpful as many
may not disclose this complication initially, but may wish to
further at another appointment. In some situations, a patient's
ay volunteer the information. It is important that, if ED is dis-
a patient, then the topic should be discussed. If it is dismissed
t may not feel comfortable in discussing it again.

This can lead to an avoidance of intimacy with their partner and relationship difficulties can develop. Psychological cause of ED may result from life
events, such as bereavement, trauma, and relationship issues/problems,
and stress at work as well as events such as childhood abuse.

Table 10.1 Differences in symptoms between physical and
psychological erectile dysfunction

	Physical ED	Psychological ED
Onset	Gradual	Sudden
Nocturnal erections	None	Yes
Early morning erections	None	Yes
Ability to achieve an erection	No	Yes
Ability to achieve an erection through masturbation	No	Yes

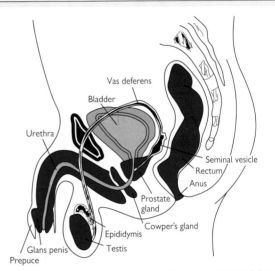

Fig. 10.1 Male genital anatomy. Reproduced from Pattman R et al (2005). *Oxford
Handbook of Genitourinary Medicine, HIV, and AIDS*, with permission from Oxford
University Press.

Further information

Eardley I, Sethia K. (2003) *Erectile dysfunction, current investigations and management,*
2nd edn. Elsevier, Amsterdam.
Feldman HA, Goldstein I, Harichriston DG, Crane KJ, McKinleny JB (1994). Impotence and its
medical and psychosexual correlates; results of the Massacheusetts Male Aging Study. *J Urology*
151, 54–61.

Causes and risk factors for erectile dysfunction

ED can be caused by alteration in any one of the following factors:
• Psychological.
• Hormonal.
• Neurological.
• Vascular.
• Penile arterial blood flow.

Conditions are associated with ED
• Diabetes.
• Heart disease.
• Liver disease (alcohol/drug misuse).
• Surgery.
• Trauma.
• Mental health issues.
• Stress.
• Psychological factors.
• Relationship difficulties.
• Medications (see Table 10.2).

Risk factors for men with diabetes developing ED
• Neuropathy (nerve damage).
• Vascular (damage to blood vessels).
• Poor glycaemic control.
• Smoking.
• Alcohol/drug misuse.
• Hyperlipidaemia.
• Hormone deficiency (low testosterone).
Some medications may also precipitate ED (see Table 10.2).

Table 10.2 Medications that may precipi

Drug class	Example
Antihypertensives	Thiazides, beta blockers, /
Anti-arrthymic	Verapamil, flecainide, pro
Antidepressant	Tricyclic antidepressants,
Antipsychotics	Phenothiazines
Lipid lowering	Statins, fibrates
Anti-convulsants	Carbamazepine, gabapenti
Alcohol	50% more likelihood of EC consumed per week
Miscellaneous	Acetazolamide, allopurinol bromocriptine, cimetidine,
	NSAIDS, oestrogens, opiat

Adapted from Cummings (2006).

Further information
Cummings M. (2006) *Managing erectile dysfunction*. Altr

Askin dysfu

Nurses ca diabetes.

Introduc
During a
can some
we may b
further ar
can help
worth no
a later co
or more b
with ED [
conducive
the numb
issues are
sideratior
patient. T
during a
to discuss
ethnic gr
may be a
It may als
their ED
guage sup

The topic
to why it
and also
to their E
fear of er

Should th
nity to as

Some me
complica
patients
discuss it
partner r
closed b
the patie

Involving partners in the discussion

For assessment and discussion of treatment options, having both partners present at a consultation for ED is very beneficial, but in the author's experience, this does not always happen. In addition, relationships should not always be assumed and some patients may not wish to have their regular partner present. Some partners may be shocked that after some time without sexual activity, successful treatments may result in the patient being able to initiate sex, so encouraging the patient to discuss treatment options with their partner should be advised. Ensuring the patient has some up-to-date written information in relation to ED can enable a patient and partner to discuss causes and treatments of ED.

Further information

Royal College of Nursing (2005). *Nurse Education in Erectile Dysfunction (NEED)*. RCN/Pfizer Ltd, London.

Assessment and investigations

A detailed description, including the onset, duration, and symptoms should be obtained [British Society of Sexual Medicine (BSSM), 2007], as well as a medical and social history. This also includes defining the problem – as Cummings (2006) notes, 10% of patients may use the definition of ED inappropriately.

Prior to consideration of treatment, an assessment of cardiac health must be carried out to determine if the heart is capable of withstanding the stress of increased physical activity. Cardiovascular fitness can be measured by using metabolic equivalent of a task (METS). This is a measure of oxygen consumption per task according to body weight. Being able to walk for 20min on the level is equivalent to 3METS, as is climbing two flights of stairs without stopping. Sexual activity with an established partner is associated with a workload of 3METS – in younger men this may be increased to 5–6METS. A certain degree of cardiovascular fitness is required for sexual activity, irrespective of the type of treatment required to make intercourse possible. A simple cardiac assessment is to ask the man if he can climb two flights of stairs or how far he can walk on the flat without becoming out of breath. The major risk in sexual activity is from the disease, not the treatment (BSSM, 2007). If a patient is unable to complete activity equivalent to 3METS then a further cardiac assessment should be required prior to commencing treatment.

Current medications (both prescribed and non-prescribed) should be reviewed. This must include checking that the patient does not take any medicines or sprays containing nitrates, as these are contraindicated when using oral medications. As many men with diabetes with ED may have purchased tablet treatment for their ED from a variety of sources, this should also be considered and asked about (the evidence of such medications being effective is very poor and often active ingredients may not be known).

Other investigations that should be considered include:
- A physical examination to assess secondary sexual characteristics.
- Blood pressure should be reviewed.
- The IIEF score can be a useful assessment tool to assess ED and assess whether treatment is working. This is a 15-point questionnaire scale described. A 5-question scale has been adapted from this (see Table 10.3). The maximum score for the IIEF-5 system is 25 and the minimum is 5. Men without erectile dysfunction have higher scores than men with erectile dysfunction.
- Other assessment tools can include Quality of Life (QOL) scores and a penile hardness scale for the patient to complete again, useful to assess if treatment is successful in obtaining erections.
- Blood tests including HBA1C, early morning testosterone levels, and sex hormone-binding globulin are required to calculate free circulating testosterone. Luteinizing hormone (LH) and follicle-stimulating hormone (FSH) blood levels should also checked. Other specific tests, such as penile tumenescence tests and Doppler ultrasonography, are not generally required unless intervention from a urology specialist is required.

Table 10.3 IIEF-5 scoring system

Over the past 6 months	Score				
	1	2	3	4	5
How do you rate your confidence that you could get and keep an erection?	Very low	Low	Moderate	High	Very high
When you had erections with sexual stimulation, how often were your erections hard enough for penetration?	Almost never or never	Much less than half the time	About half the time	Much more than half the time	Almost always or always
During sexual intercourse, how often were you able to maintain your erection after you had penetrated (entered) your partner?	Almost never or never	Much less than half the time	About half the time	Much more than half the time	Almost always or always
During sexual intercourse how difficult was it to maintain your erection to the completion of intercourse?	Extremely difficult	Very difficult	Difficult	Slightly difficult	Not difficult
When you attempted sexual intercourse, how often was it satisfactory for you?	Almost never or never	Much less than half the time	About half the time	Much more than half the time	Almost always or always

The IIEF-5 score is the sum of questions 1–5. The lowest score is 5 and the highest score 25.

Reprinted by permission from Rosen et al. (1999).

Further information

British Society for Sexual Medicine (2007). *Guidelines on the Management of Erectile Dysfunction.* Available at ⌨ www.bssm.org.uk

Cummings M. (2006) *Managing erectile dysfunction.* Altman Publishing, St. Albans.

Rosen RC, Cappelleri JC, Smith MD, Lipsky J, Peña BM. (1999) Development and evaluation of an abridged, 5-item version of the International Index of Erectile Function (IIEF-5) as a diagnostic tool for erectile dysfunction. *Int J Impotence Res* **11**, 319–26. Available at ⌨ http://www.nature.com/ijir/index.html.

Treatment of erectile dysfunction: overview and oral medications

Overview

When discussing treatments for ED, lifestyle factors in relation to diabetes are significant. Maximizing glycaemic control and regular physical activity can help in restoring erectile function. The effects of alcohol, smoking, and recreational drugs are all factors that will cause ED and should be advised about, but should not preclude treatment (Cummings 2006).

Schedule 11

Under Schedule 11 of NHS regulations for prescribing drug treatments for ED, prescribers can prescribe treatments for ED under a list of medical conditions, which includes diabetes. The schedule recommends 4 treatments a month for NHS patients, but also states that the amount a prescriber can give is at his/her clinical judgment of the patient on an individual basis.

Oral medications.

For most men with diabetes, unless contraindicated, oral medication is the preferred treatment option.

Types of drugs

These drugs are the phosphodiesterase type 5 (PDE5) inhibitors sildenafil, tadalafil, and vardenafil (BNF, 2008) These drugs work by enhancing the neurotransmitter chemicals in the parasympathetic nervous system causing relaxation and tumescence within the penile blood supply. (Cummings, 2008). All have similar modes of action, side effects, and contraindications, but differ in their response times and 'window of opportunity' for their clinical effectiveness (see Table 10.4).

PDE5s

All PDE5s are contraindicated in patients receiving nitrate medications following recent stroke, myocardial infarction, and unstable angina, or in patients with a previous history of non-arteritic anterior ischaemic optic neuropathy, hypotension (a systolic bp below 90mmHg) or in whom patients where sexual activity is inadvisable (BNF, 2008).

Patient information

Patients should be advised that sexual arousal is required for the drugs to be effective. At least 8 doses of the drug at maximum dose should be considered to assess effectiveness and, if one drug is not effective, switching to another PDE5s can be considered. (American Urology Association 2006). Tadalafil has a longer opportunity of an erection occurring as it can effect an erection for up to 48h after the drug is taken. Some studies demonstrate that some men prefer tadalafil for this reason (BSSM, 2007). This drug can also be used as a trial of therapy by using 2 or 3 times per week, which some men prefer as it allows them to regain some spontaneity in relation to sexual activity over the shorter-acting preparations (Mirone et al, 2005; BSSM, 2007).

Effectiveness

Generally, the efficiency rates for the 3 drugs are very similar (BSSM, 2007). There is no evidence that one PDE5 is more effective over another one (American Urological Association, 2006). Personal choice by the patient over which PDE5 to use according to 'the window of opportunity' each drug presents is appropriate.

Coronary events

After a coronary event, diabetic men are often prescribed GTN sprays, which preclude the use of PDE5s. Men who never use these sprays and who present with ED should have these treatments assessed either by their GP or cardiologist, and if appropriate, with agreement between patient and HCP, these GTN sprays may be discontinued to enable them to use PDE5s (BSSM, 2007).

Table 10.4 Oral medications with side effects

Treatment	Formulation and doses available	Contraindications	Advice regarding food	When before sex to take it	How long it is effective for	Common side effects
Tadalafil (CIALIS)	Tablet 10 and 20 mg	Nitrates. Avoid concurrent use with alpha blockers	Can be taken with or without food	At least 30min	Up to 36h	Headache. Dyspepsia
Vardenafil (Levitra)	Tablet 5, 10 and 20mg	Nitrates. Avoid alpha blockers for 6h after vardenafil	Can be taken with or without food. If taken with a high fat meal it may take longer to work	~30–60min	Up to 4–5h	Headaches. Flushes
Sildenafil (Viagra)	Tablet 25, 50, and 100mg	Nitrates. Avoid alpha blockers for 4h after sildenafil	May take longer to work with food	~1h	Up to 4–5h	Headaches. Flushes

Further information

American Urological Association (2006) *Management of erectile dysfunction*. Available at ▣ www.avaent.org/guidelines

British National Formulary (March 2008). *Drugs for Erectile Dysfunction*. Available at ▣ www.bnf.org.uk

British Society for Sexual Medicine (2007). *Guidelines on the management of erectile dysfunction*. Available at ▣ www.bssm.org.uk

Cummings M. (2006). *Managing erectile dysfunction*. Altman Publishing, St. Albans.

Cummings M. (2008). Assessment and treatment options for erectile dysfunction. *Prescriber* **19**(8), 49–57.

Mirone V, Costa P, Damber JE, et al. (2005) An evaluation of an alternative dosing regimen with tadalafil, 3 times/week, for men with erectile dysfunction: SURE study in 14 European countries. *Eur Urol* **47**(6), 846–54.

Treatment of erectile dysfunction: other treatment options

If PDE5s are contraindicated, not effective, or not tolerated, other treatment options include vacuum pumps, alprostadil (intracavernosal or intraurethral) medication, and penile implants (Cummings, 2008).

Vacuum pumps

Vacuum pumps are available on prescription under schedule 11. These pumps work by a plastic cylinder being applied over the penis and drawing air out of the cylinder using a hand pump attached to the cylinder. This creates a vacuum effect, allowing blood to enter the corpora cavernosa, so causing an erection. The erection is maintained by applying a constriction ring to the base of the penis. Explanation, demonstration, and regular practice are required for them to be effective. They should be used with caution with patients with bleeding disorders or for patients using anticoagulation therapy. Some patient's partners find vacuum pumps unacceptable as the erections produced can be cold and the penis discoloured. They can be used as an exerciser to help draw blood into the penis and can help restore confidence in men, especially if oral medication has been ineffective.

Alprostadil

Alprostadil injections and intraurethral alprostadil are also effective treatments, but both require explanation and careful teaching of injection technique with dose titration until erections occur. Alprostadil injections involve injecting into the side of the penis into the corpora cavernosal tissue. Intraurethral alprostadil is delivered as a small pellet of the drug inserted into the urethra via an introducer. Common side effects of alprostadil therapy include penile pain, trauma to the penis, hypotension and dizziness, and the potential for the rare side effect of an erection occurring that does not subside after 4h (priapism). Patients who are prescribed alprostadil injections should be made aware that they should seek medical help if this occurs – without treatment erections can become very painful and damage to the penis can occur. However, all these treatments can have effective results.

Surgical implants

Surgical implants: whilst these are not a first or second line treatment, surgical implants can be used to treat ED in patients in whom other treatment is not successful. This surgery involves the insertion of penile inflatable prosthesis.

Treatment in the case of hormone deficiency

Hormone deficiency in the adult male becomes more common with increasing age (Morales et al, 2004), but its management remains controversial (BSSM, 2007). As well as sexual dysfunction, deficiency is associated with osteoporosis and dyslipidaemia, Type 2 diabetes, metabolic syndrome, and depression (BSSM, 2007). The evidence for treating men with low testosterone levels in the absence of clinical hypogonadal features is still inconclusive, but if the levels of testosterone are low and the patient complains of low libido, together with unsuccessful treatment then referral to a consultant endocrinologist is recommended.

Psychosexual therapy

This can be useful as most men will have some emotional issues or anxiety regarding their performance, even if the cause is organic. If ED is due to a psychological cause then counselling and psychosexual therapy should be the first line of treatment before considering other treatment options.

Further information

Cummings M. (2008). Assessment and treatment options for erectile dysfunction. *Prescriber* **19**(8), 49–57.

Rosen RC, Riley A, Wagner G, et al (1997). The International Index of Erectile Dysfunction (IIEF); a multidimensional scale for the assessment of erectile dysfunction. *Urology* **49**, 822–9.

Eardley I, Sethia K. (2003) *Erectile dysfunction, current investigations and management*, 2nd edn. Elsevier, Amsterdam.

Morales A, Bucat J, Groven LJ, et al. (2004). Endocrine aspects of sexual dysfunction in men. *J Sex Med* **1**, 69–81.

British Society for Sexual Medicine. *Guidelines on the management of erectile dysfunction*. Available at ⌨ www.bssm.org.uk

Useful patient resources

Leaflets

Sex and Diabetes. Available from Diabetes UK at: ▣ www.diabetes.org.uk

Useful sources of information

The Impotence Association, PO Box 10296, London SW17 9WH, UK. Tel: 020 8767 7791.
Available at: ▣ www.impotence.org.uk

The Sexual Dysfunction Association, Suite 301 Emblem House, London Bridge Hospital, 27 Tooley
Street, London SE1 2PR, UK. Helpline 08707743571. Available at: ▣ www.sda.uk.net

Relate, Herbert Gray College, Little Church Street, Rugby CV21 3AP, UK. Tel: 0845 1304016.
Available at: ▣ www.relate.org.uk

Useful sites

BBC Relationships Advice ▣ www.bbc.co.uk/relationships
Sort ED in 10. ED advice ▣ www.sortedin10.co.uk

Chapter 11

Stages of life and diabetes

Stages of life and diabetes: overview

Reaction to the diagnosis of diabetes is contingent on physiological, psychological, and experiential factors. Any or all of these factors may affect the individual's ability to cope with the condition. Physiologically, the combination of diabetes, an endocrine condition, and other endocrine fluctuations, such as childhood growth spurts, puberty, pregnancy, and the menopause, all impact on the difficulties of maintaining optimal glucose control. Psychological and experiential influences, such as family members having the disease and their ability to cope, and other relatives who may have suffered the long-term complications, may impact on attitudes towards blood glucose (BG) management. Age at diagnosis, duration of the condition, and physiological adjustments to different stages of life and life events bring with them adjustments and turmoil that are factors shaping day-to-day confidence in self-management.

Adolescence

Teenage years are generally associated with rebellion and a desire for greater independence, as the physical and social transitions from childhood to adulthood takes place. This creates many challenges for parents and healthcare professionals (HCP) supporting families during these years of physiological and psychological change. There is evidence of an increase in diabetes-related emergency admissions to hospital for young people, with Type 1 diabetes, during adolescence.

During these years parents are tackling the difficult transition of handing over the responsibilities of daily control of diabetes to their offspring. Some adolescent rebellion manifests itself in manipulative behaviour regarding continuing with the regimen of giving regular injections of insulin and monitoring BG levels. This is often an additional cause of family conflict at this challenging time in parenting.

Protocols are required to manage the transition from services designed for children to the provision of adult services, including call/recall to prevent young people being lost to the service.

Standards 5 and 6 of the NSF (2003) for diabetes cite as the aim of care delivery:

> To ensure that the special needs of children and young people with diabetes are recognized and met, thereby ensuring that, when they enter adulthood, they are in the best of health and able to manage their own day to day diabetes care effectively. (p. 27)

Aims of diabetes care delivery during adolescence

- Educational input and discussion tailored to the individual's needs and abilities.
- To promote understanding of implications and individual choice regarding regimes of monitoring, dose adjustments, and insulin delivery.
- Promotion of physical and psychological wellbeing.
- Normal growth and development.
- Avoidance of preventable diabetes-related hospitalization.
- Achievement of good glycaemic control to limit the risk of long-term microvascular complications.
- Regular screening for the detection of complications, NICE (2004) guidelines for young people aged 11–17 years suggests screening for:
  - coeliac disease at diagnosis and at least every 3 years thereafter
  - thyroid disease at diagnosis and annually thereafter
  - annually for retinopathy from the age of 12 years
  - annually for microalbuminuria from the age of 12 years
  - blood pressure annually from the age of 12 years.
- Successful integration into:
  - school, college, and university life
  - social life
  - working life.

Insulin regimes

At this time of change an intensive insulin therapy, either multiple injection or continuous insulin infusion via a pump provides greater flexibility for:

- Timing meals.
- Timing injections or bolus delivery.
- Adjustments to suit carbohydrate intake, exercise, and BG levels.
- Monitoring.
- Spontaneity for sporting or social activities.

Monitoring glycaemic control
(see 📖 Chapter 7, pp. 119–160)

Home BG monitoring, result recording, and interpretation and response to the results are essential to enable the young person with diabetes to take control of their treatment. Pre-prandial BG should be between 4–8mmol/l and post-prandial below 10mmol/l HbA1c less than 7.5% (without frequent disabling hypoglycaemia; NICE 2004).

Further information

NICE Diabetes Guidance 🖥 www.diabetes.nhs.uk/reading-room/nice

Department of Health (2003) *The National Service Framework for Diabetes (Standards)* HMSO, London.

NICE (2004) *Diagnosis and management of Type 1 diabetes in children, young people and adults.* NICE, London.

Contraception: overview

Important points to remember

- The full range of contraceptive methods is normally suitable for the diabetic woman, but use of combined oral contraception for the woman who is normotensive, whose diabetes control is stable, and has no signs of complications, should be accompanied by regular diabetic control surveillance.
- Any discussion about contraception is both sensitive and highly personal to individual women and their partners.
- You need to be knowledgeable about the local services available to best meet the woman's needs.
- Contraception and sexual health are continually developing and, unless you work in the specialty, it is difficult to give anything other than general information and leaflets. It is far better to refer her to the local contraception (family planning) service for specialist management.
- Ensure that you have up-to-date information on the full range of contraceptive methods available, clinics in the locality, access to relevant, appropriate websites, and useful books that might help.
- Allow plenty of time for discussion and ensure an appropriate environment to maintain confidentiality and encourage a relaxed discussion.
- Remember that, to be effective, the chosen contraception must be used properly and, therefore, acceptable to the woman and, ideally, her partner.

Contraceptive methods

Hormonal
- Combined oestrogen and progesterone:
  - oral combined pill
  - contraceptive patch.
- Progesterone only:
  - oral progesterone only pill
  - injectables
  - implant
  - intrauterine system.

Non-hormonal
- Intrauterine device.
- Barrier:
  - male condom
  - female condom
  - diaphragm and cervical cap.
- Natural:
  - breast feeding (lactational amenorrhoea)
  - fertility awareness.
- Surgical:
  - male sterilization
  - female sterilization.

Emergency contraception

How does it work?

These methods inhibit implantation, should unwanted conception have occurred. It is vital that the woman clearly understands that this relates only to the immediately preceding 72h, even if there are multiple episodes of intercourse within this period. Any episodes in the current cycle occurring prior to this 72h period may have already resulted in pregnancy and will render emergency contraception totally ineffective.

There are two methods:
- **Oral progesterone preparation:** levonorgestrel, commonly known as the 'morning after pill', although this terminology should be discouraged, as it is misleading.
- **Copper intrauterine device.**

The emergency contraception pill

- The pill has maximum efficacy of 99.6% if taken within 24h and 98.9% at 72h.
- Treatment may be repeated in any menstrual cycle, if necessary.
- There is no evidence of any effect on the foetus if taken in early pregnancy.
- If any doubt about whether pregnancy is possible, a pregnancy test should be carried out prior to administration.
- Side effects are virtually none.
- The period may be heavier, but should occur at the expected time.
- Follow-up is normally after the expected date of the next period, normally about 3 weeks, to ensure that the period has occurred or, if not, a pregnancy test is undertaken.

Intrauterine device (IUD)

- It can be inserted up to 5 days after unprotected intercourse or up to 5 days after the earliest calculation of the day of ovulation.
- Usually a copper IUD is inserted and removed following the next period.
- If the woman decides that she wishes to keep the IUD as a long-term method of contraception, one with a life span of up to 10 years can be inserted.
- Follow-up is normally 1 week after next expected period, to check that the woman has had a normal period or, if she has not, to undertake a pregnancy test.

Emergency contraception for women with diabetes

It may be advisable for a woman with diabetes to use emergency contraception if she has poor diabetes control, or active eye or renal complications that would deteriorate in pregnancy.

Further information

Useful websites

Faculty of Family Planning and Reproductive Health. Available at: 🖳 http://www.ffprhc.org.uk
International Planned Parenthood Federation. Available at: 🖳 http://www.ippf.org
The Family Planning Association. Available at: 🖳 http://www.fpa.org.uk
World Health Organization. Available at: 🖳 http://www.who.int/topics/family_planning/en/

Books

Everett S. (2004) *Handbook of contraception and reproductive sexual health*, 2nd edn. Bailliere Tindall, London.
Guillebaud J. (2004a) *Contraception: your questions answered*, 4th edn. Churchill Livingstone, Edinburgh.
Guillebaud J. (2004b) *Contraception today*, 5th edn. Martin Dunitz, London.
NICE (2005) *Long acting reversible contraception*, clinical guideline. RCOG Press, London.
NICE (2008) *Diabetes in pregnancy*, clinical guideline 63. NICE, London.

Pre-conception care

To avoid or minimize the complications and risks to mother and baby of poorly regulated BG levels in pregnancy, it is important that the woman has effective contraception, appropriate BG control, and evidence-based information about the risks prior to conception. Preconception care and good BG control before and during pregnancy can reduce the risks (CEMACH 2006).

Women with Type 1 and Type 2 diabetes have high risk pregnancies compared with the general maternity population

Their babies are:
- Five times more likely to be stillborn.
- Three times more likely to die in the first month of life.
- Twice as likely to have major congenital abnormality.
- Five times as likely to deliver before 37 weeks.
- Twice as likely to be over 4kg at birth.
- Ten times more likely to have Erb's palsy (CEMACH 2005)

All women of childbearing age with diabetes should receive the following information:
- The risks associated with pregnancy.
- Good BG control before and during pregnancy offers the best chance of decreasing the risks.
- HbA1c should be <7%.
- Home BG tests should not be higher than 5.5mmol/l before meals and 7.7mmol/l 2h after meals (Diabetes UK 2002)
- Effective and reliable contraception is important to avoid an unplanned pregnancy.
- She should contact her diabetes care team if considering becoming pregnant.

Women who wish to become pregnant

- Check HbA1c.
- Refer the woman as soon as possible to a preconception diabetes clinic or to the diabetes care team.
- Review current medication:
  - discontinue ACE inhibitors and commence methyldopa if an antihypertensive is required
  - discontinue statins
  - if on oral hypoglycaemic agents, change to insulin under the supervision of the diabetes care team
  - continue contraception.
- Monitor BG more frequently (at least 4 times a day) as advised by the diabetes care team.
- Prescribe folic acid 5mg daily, to continue until the woman is 12 weeks pregnant, to minimize the risk of neural tube defect in the first few weeks of pregnancy.
- Offer smoking cessation advice, if appropriate.
- Explain the benefits of breast feeding (including improved BG control and easier maternal weight loss after birth).

Further information

Confidential Enquiry into Maternal and Child Health (CEMACH) (2005) *Pregnancy in women with Type 1 and Type 2 diabetes in 2002–2003, England, Wales and Northern Ireland.* RCOG Press, London. Available at: 🖳 www.cemach.org.uk

Confidential Enquiry into Maternal and Child Health (CEMACH) (2006) *Important information for general practitioners and the primary care team. women with Type 1 and Type 2 diabetes.* CEMACH, London. Available at: 🖳 www.cemach.org.uk

Diabetes UK Care Recommendations (2002) *Preconception care for women with diabetes.* Available at: 🖳 www.diabetes.org.uk/infocentre/carerec/precencept.htm

Diabetes during pregnancy

The classification of diabetes during pregnancy falls into three forms:
- Type 1 diabetes, which is present prior to pregnancy.
- Type 2 diabetes.
- Gestational diabetes (GDM) or impaired glucose tolerance, which arises as a result of pregnancy and then resolves after the birth. The incidence is between 3 and 12% of the pregnant population. Overt diabetes will develop in 20–30% of sufferers within 5 years (Peters et al., 1996).

Non-diabetic pregnant women are offered a glucose challenge screen to detect GDM if any two of the following risk factors are present:
- Glycosuria on two occasions on testing at an antenatal visit (early morning sample).
- History of diabetes in a close relative.
- Obesity, BMI >27.
- Previous baby weighing more than 4.5kg.
- Previous unexplained perinatal death.
- Previous baby with congenital malformations.
- Unexplained severe polyhydramnios (excess amniotic fluid in the uterus).

Maternal complications that might arise in the pregnant diabetic client

These are related to poorly-controlled glucose levels in the maternal serum:
- Urinary tract infection.
- Vaginal infection.
- Polyhydramnios.
- Pregnancy-induced hypertension.
- Foetal macrosomia leading to shoulder dystocia.

Foetal complications
- Congenital abnormality is 4 times higher than in non-diabetics.
- Prematurity associated with delayed lung maturity.
- Perinatal death (due to the above conditions).
- 1:100 risk of the child itself becoming diabetic.

Carbohydrate metabolism during pregnancy (non-diabetic)

- Pregnancy itself is said to be diabetogenic as a result of changes due to the action of the pregnancy hormones.
- The foetal/placental unit alters glucose metabolism in the following ways:
  - from the 10th week fasting blood sugar progressively falls from 4 to 3.6mmol/l
  - the placenta produces a hormone called human placental lactogen (HPL), which increases the maternal tissue resistance to insulin
  - blood glucose levels therefore are higher after meals and remain so for longer than in the non-pregnant state.
- More insulin is required by the body and output of insulin in the pancreas increases by 3–4 times the normal rate.
- Extra demands on the pancreatic beta cells precipitate glucose intolerance or overt diabetes in women whose capacity to produce insulin was only just adequate prior to pregnancy (gestational diabetes).
- Utilization of fat stores results in raised free fatty acid and glycerol levels, making the woman more readily ketotic.

Management of diabetes/gestational diabetes

If the mother is already diabetic, her insulin requirements will be increased during pregnancy and her pregnancy will need to be monitored carefully (RCOG, 2008).

If it is safely achievable, women with diabetes should aim to keep fasting BG between 3.5 and 5.9mmol/l and 1h post-prandial BG below 7.8mmol/l during pregnancy.

Women with Type 2 diabetes may form the largest population of pre-pregnancy diabetics and be exposed to the same levels of risk related to pregnancy outcomes. Their condition may, indeed, be diagnosed for the first time during pregnancy due to screening for GDM. Careful monitoring of glycaemic control, and provision of insulin as a replacement or in addition to metformin therapy could improve outcomes.

For women who develop GDM a careful assessment of their insulin needs is required and therapy commenced in accordance with the need to control BG levels in the prescribed range.

Women with insulin-treated diabetes should be advised of the risks of hypoglycaemia and hypoglycaemia unawareness in pregnancy, particularly in the first trimester. During pregnancy, women with insulin-treated diabetes should be provided with a concentrated glucose solution and women with Type 1 diabetes should also be given glucagon. Women and their partners or other family members should be instructed in their use.

Further information

Peters RK, Kjos SL, Xiang A, Buchanan TA. (1996) Long-term diabetogenic effect of single pregnancy in women with previous gestational diabetes mellitus. *Int J Gynecol Obstet* **54**, 213.

RCOG (2008) *Diabetes in pregnancy: management of diabetes and its complications from preconception to the postnatal period.* Commissioned by the National Institute for Health and Clinical Excellence March 2008. RCOG Press, London.

General principles of care for women with diabetes in pregnancy

Preconception care

- Ensure as much as possible that pregnancies are planned.
- Early booking (before the 10th week of pregnancy).
- Joint care with an endocrinologist specializing in diabetes.
- Blood sugar profiles every 2 weeks and glycosylated haemoglobin monthly.
- Prevention of excessive maternal weight gain and early referral to dietetic services.
- Healthcare professionals should be aware that the rapid-acting insulin analogues (aspart and lispro) have advantages over soluble human insulin during pregnancy and should consider their use.
- Pregnant women with pre-existing diabetes should be offered retinal assessment by digital imaging with mydriasis using tropicamide following their first antenatal clinic appointment and again at 28 weeks if the first assessment is normal. If any diabetic retinopathy is present, an additional retinal assessment should be performed at 16–20 weeks. If retinal assessment has not been performed in the preceding 12 months, it should be offered as soon as possible after the first contact in pregnancy in women with pre-existing diabetes. If retinopathy is found during pregnancy, patients will require follow-up after delivery for at least 6 months.
- If renal assessment has not been undertaken in the preceding 12 months in women with pre-existing diabetes, it should be arranged at the first contact in the pregnancy. If serum creatinine is abnormal (120μmol/l or more) or if total protein excretion exceeds 2g/day, referral to a nephrologist should be considered (eGFR should not be used during pregnancy). Thromboprophylaxis should be considered for women with proteinuria above 5g/day (macroalbuminuria).
- Careful screening for urinary tract and vaginal infection, with prompt treatment.
- Discuss the need for a foetal anomaly scan in light of the increased risk of malformations.
- Careful monitoring of foetal growth by regular ultrasound scans.
- At 36 weeks gestation, a discussion should take place with the mother regarding the mode of delivery and the options available.
  A recommendation of induction of labour or elective caesarean section should be made should the maternal or foetal condition warrant this.

Diabetes and intrapartum care

The nurse may meet pregnant women in the delivery suite who experience pre-existing Type 1 diabetes (insulin-dependant), pre-existing diabetes Type 2 (controlled by medication/diet, but requiring insulin during pregnancy), or gestational diabetes (which develops in pregnancy and may or may not require insulin) and which usually resolves following delivery.

The lead professional for a woman with diabetes experiencing childbirth is the obstetric consultant. The role of the midwife during intrapartum care is to help implement the plan of care that should be developed antenatally in conjunction with the woman, partner, and multidisciplinary team.

The midwife should liaise with the team and ensure all are aware of the woman's progress (NMC 2004).

An appropriately trained registered nurse may help monitor and support the woman's medical needs, where high dependency staffing permits. However, the midwife remains responsible for providing midwifery care and should remain with the woman throughout labour and birth (NMC 2004, Medforth et al 2006).

Diabetes may cause complications antenatally that increase the risks to the mother and foetus during intrapartum care. For example:
- Pre-term labour is more common (Medforth et al). Women with Types 1 and 2 diabetes are 5 times more likely to give birth before 37 weeks than women without diabetes (CEMACH 2005).
- There may be excess water/liquor around the foetus *in utero* (polyhydramnios). Consequently, the foetus may take up an unstable/unusual position, e.g. the cord may present first or prolapse into the vagina when the membranes (bag of waters) rupture. Also, following birth, the over-stretched uterine muscle may contract less effectively to stem the flow of blood at the placental site and post-partum haemorrhage may result.
- A large baby (macrosomic or >4kg) may result in the shoulders becoming impacted during the birth (shoulder dystocia). Birth injury to the baby may occur (commonly Erb's palsy, damage to the upper braxial plexus) or, in the worst cases, brain damage or death/stillbirth.
- Pregnancy-induced hypertension is more common and frequently more severe than in the general maternity population, and this may cause complications in labour.
- If the diabetes is not well controlled intrauterine death or stillbirth may ensue.
- Major congenital anomalies are twice as likely to occur when diabetes is present (CEMACH 2005). Usually, they are excluded antenatally by ultrasound scan.

Obstetricians usually recommend a proactive approach to timing and mode of delivery in order to minimize these risks. 2 out of 3 pregnant women with Type 1 and 2 diabetes deliver by caesarean section.

It is **recommended** that pregnant women with diabetes and with a normally grown foetus should be offered elective birth after 38 weeks gestation (NICE 2008). Labour should be induced or a caesarean section performed.

The reason for intervention is to prevent stillbirth and shoulder dystocia associated with foetal macrosomia at term. The timing of 38 weeks is to avoid the risk of respiratory distress syndrome due to an early birth.

Nevertheless, each woman should be treated as an individual. She should be given informed choice. When the diabetes is well controlled and the foetus is normally grown, the woman may wish to go to term and into labour spontaneously. This is acceptable with appropriate monitoring (Arulkumaran et al 2004).

Further information

Arulkumaran S, Symonds IM, Fowlie A. (2004). *Oxford Handbook of Obstetrics and Gynaecology.* Oxford University Press, Oxford.

Confidential Enquiry into Maternal and Child Health (CEMACH) (2005). *Pregnancy in women with Type 1 and 2 diabetes in 2002–2003, England, Wales and Northern Ireland.* RCOG Press, London. Available at: 🖳 www.cemach.org.uk

Medforth J, Battersby S, Evans M, Marsh B, Walker A. (2006). *Oxford Handbook of Midwifery.* Oxford University Press, Oxford.

National Institute for Clinical Excellence (NICE) (2008). *Diabetes in pregnancy, management of diabetes and its complications from preconception to the postnatal period,* Guideline 63. NICE, London. Available at: 🖳 www.nice.org.uk

Nursing and Midwifery Council (NMC) (2004). *Midwives rules and standards,* Rule 6. NMC, London. Available at: 🖳 www.nmc-uk.org

Sheffield Teaching Hospitals (STH) NHS Trust (2008). *The labour ward guidelines.* STH, Sheffield.

Vaginal birth

The aim of care is to promote maternal and foetal wellbeing, to support the family to begin to develop effective parenting, and to optimize the normal childbirth experience for the woman whilst ensuring safety.

The activities of the midwife

These include:

- Careful communication with the woman and listening to obtain a history, develop a trusting relationship, and to recognize the woman's ordinary and individual needs.
- Assessment of maternal vital signs, fluid balance, and wellbeing, inspection and palpation of the woman's abdomen to monitor the strength, length, and frequency of contractions, and position, presentation, descent, and wellbeing of the foetus.
- Monitoring the woman's progress in labour, recognizing latent and active phases, and observing for deviation from the normal.
- Discussing coping strategies for labour, pain management choices, and anaesthesia. These should initially be discussed with the woman in the third trimester of pregnancy. When a women has diabetes, epidural anaesthesia may be offered, but the woman's preferences should be respected.
- Caring and support for the woman and family during the actual birth of the baby. The obstetric registrar and paediatrician should be available to help in case of maternal post-partum haemorrhage, foetal compromise, or shoulder dystocia.
- Attentive assessment of the mother immediately after the birth. An intramuscular injection of oxytocin may be given to promote uterine contractions and facilitate placental delivery.
- Inspection and any suturing of perineum.
- Assessment of the newborn and ensuring the baby is kept warm by skin-to-skin contact with the mother. Feeding should be promptly established and the neonate treated as high risk for hypoglycaemia.
- Detailed documentation of care given.

The aim of diabetic care during labour and childbirth is to maintain the maternal BG in the range of 4–7mmol/l. This has been shown to reduce the incidence of neonatal hypoglycaemia and to reduce foetal distress (NICE 2008):

- BG should be assessed every 30min until stable, then hourly. When the 4–7mmol/l range is not maintained iv dextrose and insulin pump is recommended.
- From the onset of active labour (regular painful contractions accompanied by dilatation of the cervix) women with Type 1 diabetes should always be advised to have iv cannulation, a dextrose infusion and an insulin pump, e.g. 500ml 10% dextrose saline + 10mmol KCl set to run at 100ml/h. An insulin pump with soluble insulin 50IU in 49.5ml normal saline is set to run according to regime. Augmented regime may be used, following obstetric review, when the BG is >17mmol/l and desired range is not achieved (see Table 11.1).

Table 11.1 Example of insulin sliding scale regime (STH 2008)

Blood glucose (mmol/l)	Insulin dose (IU/h), standard regime	Insulin dose (IU/h), augmented regime
<4	0	0
4–5	1	2
6–7	2	4
8–12	3	6
13–17	4	8
>17	6	12

- Blood glucose levels can be erratic in labour because there is a great need for energy, which helps facilitate the rhythmic contractions of the uterine muscle.
- Occasionally, dehydration or infection may lead to a high BG and ketoacidosis. The foetus is very vulnerable to ketoacidosis and may quickly die. The midwife should be vigilant, and assess fluid balance and test all urine for ketones. Venous blood samples should be obtained to assess urea, electrolytes, and bicarbonate. The foetal heart should be monitored continuously throughout labour using cardiotocography (CTG). The midwife should be expert on the interpretation of the CTG. Any deviation from normal should be reported to the obstetric registrar.
- Following the birth of the baby, once the mother is free from nausea and has a stable BG the iv insulin regime may be discontinued:
  - in Type 1 diabetes the mother may be encouraged to have normal insulin and diet
  - in Type 2 diabetes the mother may return to her pre-pregnancy regime of monitoring BG, and medication or diet
  - in gestational diabetes, the BG usually returns to normal.

Further information

National Institute for Clinical Excellence (NICE) (2008). *Diabetes in pregnancy, management of diabetes and its complications from preconception to the postnatal period*, Guideline 63. NICE, London.

Sheffield Teaching Hospitals (STH) NHS Trust (2008). *The labour ward guidelines*. STH, Sheffield.

Induction of labour

Women who have diabetes and require induction of labour should be given priority in the delivery suite and should experience vigilant care from the midwife.

- Normal diet and insulin should be given on the day prior to induction. During the evening, prostaglandin gel or tablet may be inserted into the vagina to 'ripen' (soften) the cervix. The foetal heart should be monitored using the CTG. Any deviations from the norm must be reported to the obstetric registrar.
- On the day of induction, the woman may take normal rapid-acting insulin and breakfast. The consultant obstetrician should review the woman's care and, if possible, the membranes holding the liquid that naturally surrounds the foetus may be artificially ruptured (ARM): a vaginal examination should be performed, and an instrument used to puncture and part the membranes palpable through the cervical os. This stimulates uterine activity and allows the midwife to visualize the liquor, which may give information about foetal wellbeing.
- Maternal BG must be monitored. A regime as shown in Table 11.1 for iv fluids and insulin sliding scale should be commenced as necessary.
- If uterine contractions have not started spontaneously a regime using iv oxytocin, which stimulates the uterus to contract, should promote cervical dilatation.
- The foetal heart should be continuously monitored throughout labour.
- The woman may progress to a vaginal birth (see 📖 p. 250).
- If progress is delayed or there is suspected foetal compromise, a decision may be taken to expedite delivery by ventouse, forceps, or caesarean section.

Emergency or elective caesarean section

- The midwife should prepare the woman for theatre, maintaining iv fluids and the insulin pump according to the sliding scale.
- Preparation should include medication given to the woman to neutralize gastric contents.
- The woman should be encouraged to wear anti-embolic stockings to reduce the risk of deep vein thrombosis.
- An explanation of the rationale for the caesarean should be given to the woman and her partner, and informed consent should be obtained. When local anaesthetic is used, the partner may accompany the woman to theatre.
- Theatre personnel should be alerted.
- In case of the need for a blood transfusion, full blood count and 'group and save' samples should be dispatched, and the results available.
- An in-dwelling catheter to the bladder is necessary. A full bladder could be damaged during the procedure. Fluid balance should be monitored.
- The anaesthetist should ensure adequate anaesthesia, usually by continuing an epidural or by siting a spinal anaesthetic, but sometimes using general anaesthesia (GA). When GA is used, the woman's BG should be monitored every 30min from induction of GA, until the baby is born and the mother fully conscious (Medforth et al 2006). This is because there is a risk of hypoglycaemia.
- The position of the mother on the operating table should be slightly left lateral to prevent the weight of the uterus causing pressure on the large abdominal blood vessels, which can impede venous return and cause fainting.
- Prophylactic antibiotics are usually given.
- Following delivery, the midwife should monitor the mother's recovery. Cord blood analysis should be used to record the condition of the infant
- As soon as is practical, the baby should be placed in skin-to-skin contact with the mother. Early feeding should be facilitated.

If the mother wishes to attempt a normal birth in the future, she should be aware that diabetes is not a contraindication to vaginal birth after caesarean section (Medforth et al 2006).

Further information

Medforth J, Battersby S, Evans M, Marsh B, Walker A (2006). *Oxford Handbook of Midwifery*. Oxford University Press, Oxford.

Postnatal care, breastfeeding, and diabetes

The aim of postnatal care is to provide holistic, woman-centred care, which facilitates adaptation to motherhood, and promotes the mother's and baby's physical and psychological wellbeing. Mothers who have diabetes will have additional needs, which will need to be addressed in order to achieve these aims. The first is assisting the mother to combine good blood sugar control, whilst coping with the demands of a new baby, and the second is the preventing, detecting, and managing neonatal hypoglycaemia in the baby.

Postnatal care

The advice given to mothers who have diabetes may vary depending upon the type of diabetes. This is particularly relevant to drug therapy (NICE, 2008).

Drug therapy

- Women with insulin-treated pre-existing diabetes should be advised to reduce their insulin immediately after birth and self-monitoring of BG should be undertaken to establish the correct dose.
- Women who have Type 2 diabetes should be advised that they can resume or continue taking metformin and glibenclamide whilst breastfeeding, but should not take any other oral hypoglycaemic agents when breastfeeding. These drugs are advised by NICE (2008), but do not have UK marketing authorization specifically for pregnant and breastfeeding women; therefore, informed consent should be obtained and documented.
- Women with gestational diabetes should be advised to discontinue hypoglycaemic medication immediately after birth.

Special consideration in the postnatal period

- Prompt and effective treatment of hypoglycaemia is important when a mother is caring for her baby. Warnings should be given to all diabetic mothers about the possibility of hypoglycaemia, especially when breastfeeding. They should be advised to eat before breastfeeding the baby or have a snack handy whilst feeding.
- Mothers who have diabetes are at an increased risk of infection and the importance of high standards of hygiene should be stressed. Mothers who are breastfeeding are at an increased risk of mastitis and *Candida albicans* (thrush), especially if their blood sugar levels are poorly controlled. Therefore, they should be informed of the symptoms of mastitis and thrush, how they can help themselves, and where help is available, e.g. midwife, health visitor, breastfeeding peer supporter, National Childbirth Trust, etc.
- Mothers who are breastfeeding may require extra carbohydrate to facilitate this. An extra 50g of carbohydrate per day has been suggested (De Swiet, 1995) and how this is achieved should be discussed with the diabetic team. However, it is best to spread these extra carbohydrates equally over the day, remembering especially to increase the supper snack to cover the night-time feeds.

Transfer and follow-up

- Women with pre-existing diabetes should be referred back to routine diabetic care.
- Women with gestational diabetes should be offered lifestyle advice on weight control, diet, and exercise. Before transfer to community care they should be offered a glucose test, which should be followed up with the offer of a fasting plasma measurement at the 6 week postnatal examination and annually thereafter (NICE, 2008). They should also be informed about the risk of gestational diabetes reoccurring in any subsequent pregnancy.

Breastfeeding

- Expectant parents should be made aware that breastfeeding may reduce the risk of their child developing the disease (Jackson, 2004).
- Expectant parents should also be informed that breastfeeding facilitates better management of diabetes and improves the mother's long-term health. This is because breastfeeding is a natural response to childbirth and the hormones responsible for lactation allow the physiological changes that follow childbirth to occur more gradually.
- Diabetic mothers may find a delay in their milk production (lactogenesis II) and the milk may not 'come in' until the fourth or fifth day post-natally. Expressing (if mother and baby are separated) or breastfeeding every 2–3h during the first few days following delivery can help reduce the delay.

Further information

De Swiet M. (1995) Medical disorders in pregnancy. In: Chamberlain, G. (ed.) *Turnbull's obstetrics*, 2nd edn. Churchill Livingstone, Edinburgh.

Jackson W. (2004) Breastfeeding and Type 1 diabetes mellitus. *Br J Midwif* **12**(3), 158–9 and 162–5.

NICE (2008) *Diabetes in pregnancy: management of diabetes and its complications from pre-conception to the postnatal period*, NICE clinical guidelines 63. NICE, London.

Preventing, detecting, and managing hypoglycaemia in the baby

Babies of mothers who have diabetes are more prone to hypoglycaemia because in intrauterine life the hypertrophic islets of Langerhans produce more insulin in response to the maternal blood sugar levels. After birth the pancreas initially continues to produce excess insulin, thus causing hypoglycaemia.

- Preparation for prevention of neonatal hypoglycaemia can commence in pregnancy with the expressing and storage of colostrum for use in the immediate postnatal period. Expression and storage of colostrum should be discussed with the hospital in the antenatal period.
- After birth the mother and baby should be kept together unless there is a clinical complication (NICE, 2008a).
- Skin-to-skin contact of mother and baby is important following birth as it will help maintain the baby's temperature and conserve energy. It can also facilitate earlier breastfeeding.
- The baby should be given its first feed as soon as possible (within 30min of birth) and then 2–3-hourly until pre-feeding BG levels are maintained at 2mmol/l or more (NICE, 2008a).
- The baby's BG levels should be monitored until stabilized. The frequency and timing of testing neonatal BG levels may vary according to hospital policies, but NICE (2008a) recommend routine testing 2–4h after birth and prior to feeds until the blood sugar levels are stabilized.
- The mother and baby should not be transferred to community care until the baby's blood sugar levels have stabilized and feeding is established.
- The mother should be given the opportunity for peer support with breastfeeding (NICE, 2008b).

Further information

NICE (2008a) *Diabetes in pregnancy: management of diabetes and its complications from pre-conception to the postnatal period*, NICE clinical guidelines 63. NICE, London.

NICE (2008b) *Improving the nutrition of pregnant and breastfeeding mothers and children in low income households*. NICE public health programme guidance 11. NICE, London.

Older people

The prevalence of diabetes rises with age as increased age is associated with increased insulin resistance and decreased beta cell function:
- 1 in 20 people in the UK aged 65 have diabetes.
- 1 in 5 people in the UK over the age of 85 have diabetes.
- Across Northern European countries 1 in 3 aged over 70 have diabetes.
- The diagnosis of diabetes may be delayed in older people with symptoms being attributed to the ageing process. Type 1 diabetes can manifest for the first time in older people. We need to be mindful of our lack of experience of caring for people with Type 1 diabetes who have been taking insulin for over half a century.

There are moral and ethical dilemmas when caring for older people who have diabetes, as the balance is struck between optimizing BG control, avoiding hypoglycaemia, preserving quality of life, and empowering patients.

Groups of older people at high risk of developing diabetes
- Those with impaired fasting glucose (IFG) or impaired glucose tolerance (IGT).
- Those with a family history of diabetes.
- Women who had gestational diabetes.
- High risk ethnic groups:
  - those from the Indian subcontinent
  - Afro-Caribbean/African
  - China
  - Aboriginal
  - Torres Strait Island people.
- Those with co-morbidities associated with diabetes.
- Those who are obese or have a large waist circumference.
- Those who are inactive.
- Those on diabetogenic medications, e.g.:
  - glucocorticoids;
  - oestrogens;
  - diuretics;
  - beta blockers and some antipsychotics.

Some issues limiting self-care and education for this age group

- Poor visual acuity and/or hearing impairment.
- Cognitive impairment.
- Depression.
- Limited access to services because of mobility issues.
- Mobility difficulties may also limit exercise choices.
- Loss of manual dexterity due to arthritis may impair insulin administration/monitoring capabilities.
- Altered expectations or beliefs of the older person.
- Involvement of informal carers and consideration of their knowledge and beliefs.
- Care home residency.

Care home residency

The European Diabetes Working Party for Older People (2001–2004) noted a high degree of variability across Europe regarding the standard of care and clinical practice offered in care homes. They cite the following barriers to good clinical practice:

- Organizational difficulties.
- Lack of clarity relating to medical and nursing roles and responsibilities.
- Funding issues.
- Lack of a coherent professional framework for delivering diabetes care.
- Poor provision of education regarding diabetes for care home staff.

Allied to these problems are the increased numbers of institutionalized older people with diabetes.

Guidelines for care of older people with diabetes who are care home residents are available in different areas and cover such issues as:

- Screening for diabetes in all new residents.
- Individualized care planning for all people with diabetes.
- Monitoring of residents who are known to have diabetes.
- Methods.
- Equipment and training of staff to use, assay, and clean equipment.
- Response to excursions outside defined monitoring parameters.
- Foot care.
- Diet and nutrition.
- Eye screening.
- Hypertension screening and monitoring.
- Drug administration, timing, and route.
- Emergency treatment for hypoglycaemia.
- Sick day rules.
- Skin care.
- Continence.
- Exercise.

Standard 12 of the NSF for Diabetes states:

> All people with diabetes requiring multi-agency support will receive integrated health and social care. (p. 5)

To achieve this for older people with diabetes poses a challenge to enhance team working and clarity of communications channels. Individualized care plans should be used (see Box 11.1).

Box 11.1 Examples of topics included in an individualized care plan

- Set and record realistic glycaemic and bp targets.
- Ensure consensus with:
  - patient
  - spouse or family
  - general practitioner
  - informal caregiver
  - community nurse
  - nurse specialist in diabetes
  - hospital specialist.
- List the frequency and nature of diabetes follow-up.
- Organize glycaemic monitoring by patient or caregiver. List any training required and record when it is carried out.
- Refer to social or community services as necessary.
- Provide evidence of advice given on:
  - stopping smoking
  - increasing exercise
  - nutrition
  - reducing alcohol intake where appropriate.
- Introduce to the principles of DESMOND or DAFNE as appropriate.

Further information

European Geriatric Medicine Society (2004) *European Diabetes Working Party for Older People 2001–2004, clinical guidelines for Type 2 diabetes mellitus*. International Academy for Nutrition and Ageing, New Mexico. Available at: ▣ http://www.eugms.org/index.php?pid=83 (accessed 30 April 2008).

Sinclair AJ, Bayer AJ. (1998) *All Wales Research in Elderly (AWARE) Diabetes Study Department of Health Report, UK Government paper 121/3040*. HMSO, London.

Sinclair AJ, Finucane P. (eds) (2001) *Diabetes in old age*, 2nd edn. John Wiley & Sons Ltd, Chichester.

Lifestyle and diabetes

Lifestyle and diabetes: overview

In order to manage diabetes successfully, it is essential that the individual fits diabetes into their lifestyle, rather than the other way round. If an individual's lifestyle becomes restricted as a result of diabetes, this can lead to frustration and resentment. In the majority of cases diabetes treatment can be tailored to the individual, whether this is an eating plan, exercise, and therapeutic treatments, such as oral hypoglycaemic agents or insulin.

As well as day-to-day lifestyle issues, such as employment and driving, there is no reason why people with diabetes cannot travel and enjoy celebrations, although these may not be daily or weekly occasions. Practical tips on how to manage diabetes in these circumstances can be helpful.

At diagnosis, individuals will often raise concerns about whether diabetes will stop them undertaking certain activities. Often reassurance that this is not the case can be given. In a number of cases, particularly in Type 2 diabetes, the diagnosis may lead to positive influences on the individual's lifestyle, enabling them to reduce their weight, be more active, and stop smoking, all of which are positive contributions that an individual can make to improve their diabetes control and lifestyle.

Exercise

The benefits of exercise or increasing physical activity for people with diabetes have been well documented. These include:
- Improvement in cardiovascular health.
- Reduction in bp.
- Improved sensitivity to insulin.
- Reduction in BG levels.
- Weight loss.
- Increase in HDL cholesterol.
- Improvements in bone density.
- Improved mental health/increased feeling of wellbeing.

The Department of Health current recommendations include the following:
- Children and young people should achieve a total of 60min of moderate intensity physical activity each day at least twice weekly.
- Adults should achieve 30min/day of moderate intensity activity on 5 or more days per week.
- The recommended activity levels can be achieved in one session or spread over shorter periods of 10min or more.
- These recommendations apply to the older person in whom it is important to maintain mobility through daily activity; this will contribute to improved health.

In order for exercise to be beneficial, the activity undertaken needs to:
- Increase the pulse rate.
- Lead to the individual feeling short of breath, but with the ability to maintain a conversation.
- Increase perspiration and skin colour.

Prior to increasing exercise or activity levels, it is essential that the individual ensures there are no other medical reasons why exercise would be prohibited.

Barriers to exercise

There are a number of perceived barriers to exercise including:
- Time.
- Cost.
- Embarrassment.
- Other medical conditions that make exercise/physical activity difficult, such as arthritis.
- Fear of hypoglycaemia.

It is essential to discuss realistic measures with individuals that will facilitate an increase in exercise/physical activity and to discuss management strategies.

Type 2 diabetes on diet/and metformin and/or glitazones

As hypoglycaemia is unlikely, no specific precautions are necessary prior to exercise.

Type 2 diabetes on diet and sulphonylureas/meglitinides

As sulphonylureas may lead to hypoglycaemia it would be beneficial to monitor BG levels before exercise to ensure BG levels are sufficient. Carrying hypoglycaemia treatment is essential, alongside an appropriate snack, to be eaten during or following exercise, particularly if the exercise is prolonged. Monitoring BG levels after exercise may be helpful for the individual to assess the impact of exercise on BG levels.

If the individual is not monitoring BG, it is recommended that they ensure they have eaten prior to exercise and carry hypo treatment as above.

Type 2 diabetes on insulin +/– oral hypoglycaemic agents

As the risk of hypoglycaemia is higher with insulin, these patients need to follow the same guidance as a person with Type 1 diabetes.

Type 1 diabetes

People with Type 1 diabetes are at greater risk of hypoglycaemia during exercise/physical activity. Therefore, management of diabetes to ensure avoidance of hypoglycaemia, either during or after exercise, is essential. This can be achieved by:

- Careful BG monitoring of levels before, during, and after exercise. This will enable the individual over time to establish the effect exercise has on BG levels.
- Based on the above results, the individual may consider reduction of insulin dose or increased food intake.
- Carrying hypoglycaemia treatment and appropriate longer-acting carbohydrate.
- Depending on the activity undertaken, hypoglycaemia may occur several hours later. Therefore, BG monitoring, particularly before bed, is recommended to avoid hypoglycaemia *nocte*.
- Avoidance of excessive alcohol on the day of strenuous exercise as this may exacerbate the delayed hypoglycaemia post-exercise.

Intensive exercise

Intensive exercise will influence BG control to varying degrees, particularly in Type 1 diabetes. There are different types of intensive exercise that vary in both duration and intensity. As a result, the management of diabetes may vary.

Different types of exercise

- **Anaerobic:** sprint running, speed climbing, sprint swimming.
  - **Mixed prolonged:** football, rugby, squash, dancing.
  - **Prolonged aerobic:** long distance running, cycling.
  - **Intense aerobic:** middle distance running, rowing, canoeing, cycling with hills/sprint finishes.

Endocrinology affects of exercise:
- No glucagon response.
- No portal insulin regulation of gluconeogenesis or ketogenesis.
- Impaired catecholamine response.
- Reversed portal/systemic insulin ratios.
- Relatively excessive background insulin levels (Gallen).

(See Fig. 12.1).

These effects will all influence BG levels and potentially the performance of the individual.

Management of diabetes during intensive exercise

Consideration needs to be given to the following:
- What is the nature, duration, and intensity of the exercise?
- How much energy is required?
- When can food be taken?
- When and how should the body stores be replenished after training and events?
- Self-monitoring BG will enable the individual to learn over time how best to manage diabetes during intensive exercise.

The individual may need to consider:
- Reducing insulin, particularly basal insulin, the night before if undertaking exercise of moderate to long duration. They may also need to reduce basal insulin on day of intensive exercise to prevent hypoglycaemia.
- Reducing rapid-acting insulin before exercise depending on intensity and duration of exercise (may not need any).
- Continuous subcutaneous insulin pumps when physically possible.
- Increasing carbohydrate before exercise if viable.
- Carrying both refined and unrefined carbohydrate, or ensuring availability.
- Keeping comprehensive record of BG levels before, during, and after exercise, carbohydrate requirements before, during, and after exercise, and a record of insulin dose changes made. This will enable the individual to plan effectively for future exercise.

Extreme sports

Some sports that are considered extreme in nature also need to consider all of the above aspects, in particular avoiding hypoglycaemia, and maintaining the safety of the individual concerned and peers who may accompany them, especially in activities such as rock/mountain climbing. Solo parachuting is not allowed, although some centres will consider tandem parachuting. Scuba diving has strict regulations and further consideration may need to be given to obtaining insurance for such activities. It is recommended that the individual contacts the national sporting bodies associated with each sport, details of which are easily found on the Internet.

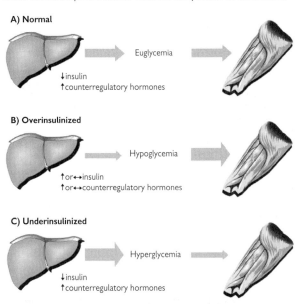

A) Normal

Euglycemia

↓insulin
↑counterregulatory hormones

B) Overinsulinized

Hypoglycemia

↑or↔insulin
↑or↔counterregulatory hormones

C) Underinsulinized

Hyperglycemia

↓insulin
↑counterregulatory hormones

Fig. 12.1 Schematic illustration of the BG response to exercise in (a) non-diabetic or ideally controlled persons with diabetes, (b) over-insulinized patients, (c) or under-insulinized patients. Reprinted with permission from the Canadian Diabetes Association © 2006.

Further information

Runsweet Diabetes and Sport 🖳 www.runsweet.com

Riddell MC, Perkins BA. (2006) Type 1 diabetes and vigorous exercise: Applications of exercise physiology to patient management *Canad J Diabet* **30**, 63–71.

Gallen I. (2006) Diabetes and sport: managing the complex interactions. *Br J Hosp Med* **67**, 634–8.

Employment

There is no reason why individuals with diabetes should not seek employment. It would be advisable, although not mandatory, for the individual to declare that they have diabetes. This may facilitate an agreement between the employer and employee regarding time off, as necessary, to attend appointments with their diabetes team. Alongside this, arrangements may be needed to enable the individual to carry out self-management of their diabetes. This may mean suitable accommodation will need to be found if BG monitoring or self-injection is not possible for the individual's immediate vicinity of their work environment.

If driving is part of the occupation certain restrictions may apply to the individual's license (see 📖 Driving: overview, p. 274).

If an ordinary vehicle license is required for the patient's occupation, this should not present any difficulties. However, if journeys are long distance, allowances may need to be made to factor in additional breaks (see 📖 Driving and diabetes: practical tips for patients, p. 276). Finally, if a company car is included in the contractual arrangements and insurance is included, it will be necessary for the employer to know that the employee has diabetes and to declare this, as failure to do so may make the insurance cover invalid.

It is against the law for an employer to discriminate against people with diabetes (Disability Discrimination Act, 1995).

Some occupations are exceptions and are not an option for individuals with diabetes. These include:
• Armed forces.
• Fire and Police service: local authorities may make exceptions, particularly if the diabetes is diagnosed during active service. The employer may consider alternative positions, as the DVLA prevent emergency vehicles being driven by individuals with diabetes.
• Airline pilots.
• Cabin crew (some airlines make exceptions).
• Train driver.
• Taxi driving: this may also be determined by local authorities.

The aim for any individual with diabetes is to ensure that the occupation chosen is suitable, and does not represent any risk to the individual themselves or to colleagues. The risks of hypoglycaemia for those on insulin or sulphonylureas must be taken into account when choosing an occupation – operating large machinery, or working in isolation or in isolated areas may not be suitable.

Individuals should be encouraged to declare their diabetes to colleagues. This may be helpful in terms of support in the work environment and may be invaluable if hypoglycaemia occurs during work time.

Some occupations require the individual to work shifts. This is possible with careful planning of carbohydrate intake and necessary adjustments to insulin therapy. A basal bolus regimen, which allows flexibility with meal times timings and doses of insulin, may be more suitable in this circumstance.

Driving: overview

The majority of individuals with diabetes are able to retain their 'till 70 driving license'. Certain restrictions apply depending on the Type of diabetes and subsequent treatment (see Table 12.1).

All drivers must be able to meet the following requirements

Be able to read in good daylight a car number plate from a distance of 20m

Therefore, individuals must inform the DVLA if:
- They are unable to meet number plate requirement.
- Any problems develop that affect the field of vision.
- Any problems develop that affect either eyes or the remaining eye, if there is sight in one eye only, or to one of both eyes.

Be able to recognize hypoglycaemia, as this represents the main hazard to safe driving

Therefore individuals must inform the DVLA if:
- Impaired awareness of hypoglycaemia develops.
- If a disabling hypoglycaemic episode occurs at the wheel.
- If frequent episodes of hypoglycaemia occur.

Limb problems

Limb problems/amputations are unlikely to prevent driving. They may be overcome by either restricting driving to certain types of vehicles, i.e. automatics or by adaptations, such as hand-operated accelerator/brake.

Therefore, individuals must inform the DVLA if complications such as neuropathy affecting sensation and/or peripheral vascular disease develop, which may cause difficulty with the safe use of foot pedals.

Individuals must also inform the DVLA if existing medical conditions deteriorate or if any other condition develops, which may affect safe driving.

Qualifying conditions

For drivers with insulin-treated diabetes who wish to apply for C1/C1E entitlement or renew entitlement to categories to drive small lorries with or without a trailer:
- No hypoglycaemic episodes requiring assistance, whilst driving within the previous 12months.
- No application will be considered, either a renewal or new application, until the diabetes has been stable for a period of at least 1month.
- Individuals must monitor BG levels at least twice daily and at times relevant to driving.
- Annual examination by a hospital consultant who specializes in diabetes, during this appointment the consultant is expected to see and review BG monitoring records.
- Individuals must have no other medical conditions, which would render them a danger when driving C1 vehicles.
- Individuals must sign an undertaking to comply with the directions of doctors treating the diabetes and to report immediately to DVLA any significant changes in their condition.

Table 12.1 DVLA restrictions

Diabetes mellitus	Group 1 entitlement (car/motorcycle)	Group 2 entitlement (VOC – LGV/PCV)
Diet alone	Need not inform the DVLA, and may retain their license till 70, unless they develop relevant disabilities, eye complications affecting visual acuity, or if insulin is required	Need not inform the DVLA, unless develop relevant disabilities, eye complications affecting visual acuity, or if insulin is required
Oral hypoglycaemic agents	Need not inform DVLA if the individual meets all the requirements set out on 📖 p. 274. Should the individual not meet all the requirements the DVLA will need to be informed, the DVLA will then make medical enquires	Drivers will be licensed unless they develop eye complications affecting visual acuity or visual fields, in which case either refusal, revocation, or short period license. If insulin treated will be refusal or revocation
Incretin-based therapy, gliptins in combination with sulphonylurea	Need not inform DVLA if the individual meets all the requirements set out on 📖 p. 274. Should the individual not meet all the requirements, the DVLA will need to be informed, the DVLA will then make medical enquires	Individual assessment
Temporary insulin treatment, e.g. in gestational diabetes, post-MI	May retain license, but should stop driving if experiencing disabling hypoglycaemia, need to notify DVLA if treatment continues for >3months	Legal bar to holding a licence while insulin treated. May re-apply when insulin treatment is discontinued
Insulin treated	Must recognize warning symptoms of hypoglycaemia and meet required visual standards. Will obtain 1, 2, or 3year licence	New applicants on insulin or existing drivers are barred in law from driving HGV or PCV vehicles from April 1991. Drivers licensed before this date are dealt with individually and licensed subject to annual consultant assessment. Exceptional cases can apply for or renew their entitlement to drive small lorries with or without trailers subject to meeting all qualifying conditions

Driving and diabetes: practical tips for patients

- Check blood sugar levels before and during the car journey (not whilst driving!).
- If blood sugar is 5.0mmol/l or less, take a snack before driving.
- Do not drive for more than 2 hours without a break, during which you test your blood sugar and a snack if necessary.
- Always carry some quick- and long-acting carbohydrate (sugary) food in your car.
- Do not miss or delay a meal or snack.
- Carry identification both on yourself and in the car. This should identify the individual as having diabetes and how it is treated.

If patients feel a hypo developing when driving, the following guidance should be given:

- **Stop** driving as soon as it is safe to do so.
- Remove the ignition key and move to the passenger seat. This is to avoid the suggestion that the person may be under the influence of drugs whilst in charge of a car.
- **Immediately** take glucose tablets, a sugary drink, or sweets.
- Follow this by taking a longer-acting carbohydrate, e.g. biscuits or crisps.
- Check blood sugar.
- Do not resume driving for 45min after blood sugar level has returned to normal.

Driving insurance

The main potential danger of diabetes and driving is hypoglycaemia. By law, motor insurance companies require the individual to declare all material facts; diabetes is considered a material fact and should be declared at the start of the policy, or when diagnosed, or during the duration of diabetes should treatment change, i.e. if insulin is commenced.

The majority of car insurance companies no longer load premiums for individuals with diabetes. If the individual feels they are being discriminated against with higher premiums, they should be advised to complain to the insurance company and, if still not satisfied, switch to another company.

Further information

DVLA website: guidelines last revised February 2008. Available at: 🖳 www.dvla.gov.uk/motoring

Police, ambulance, and health service vehicle driver licensing

Drivers with insulin-treated diabetes are not permitted to drive emergency vehicles. This takes into account of the difficulties for the individual, regardless of whether they may appear to have exemplary glycaemic control, in adhering to the monitoring processes required when responding to an emergency situation.

Travel

Where possible, travelling and holidays should be planned in advance. This will facilitate the following aspects of diabetes and travel to be taken into consideration.

Vaccinations

Individuals should be advised to find out which vaccinations are required for their proposed destination. Occasionally, minor side effects can occur and it is best to have these 4–6 weeks prior to travelling.

Travel insurance

Travel insurance is vital. Individuals should inform their insurance company and ensure that the package provides adequate cover. This should include emergency transport home if necessary. If a new policy is required, it is essential to declare all pre-existing medical conditions, failure to do so may make the insurance invalid and a claim refused. The European Health Insurance Card (EHIC) will ensure the individual has easy access to health care in the European Country Union. This should be carried in conjunction with travel insurance as it will not cover repatriation home and may not cover all health care costs in the EU.

Equipment

General advice includes:
- Taking twice as much diabetes medication as needed, including spare insulin pens, syringes if used, tablets. This should be split between passengers in case one set of luggage is lost.
- A cool bag for storing insulin if visiting a hot climate.
- Blood glucose monitoring equipment, including adequate strips and spare batteries. Individuals need to be aware that high altitudes, heat, and humidity can sometimes affect meters and may give false readings.
- Treatment for hypoglycaemia, including glucagon injection.
- Carbohydrate snacks for follow-up treatment of hypoglycaemia or for snacks if meals are delayed.
- Ketostix® in case of illness.
- Ensure diabetes identification, e.g. card or jewellery.
- A first aid kit including pain killers, antihistamines, insect repellents, anti-diarrhoea tablets, wound and blister kit, dressings, and plasters.
- A letter from either the GP or hospital clinic, confirming the individual has diabetes and needs to carry diabetes equipment.
- A list of all current medication.

Travelling with insulin

Although security restrictions prevent many items being carried on board, it is possible for insulin to be carried in hand luggage. A letter advising security staff of the need to carry diabetes equipment is advisable. Only 50ml of insulin may be carried and should be placed in a clear plastic bag. For the majority of travellers, this is sufficient in quantity as it equates to 5000units of insulin. Insulin should never be placed in the hold of the plane where it is likely to freeze. Therefore, for holidays of longer duration requiring more insulin than 5000units; arrangement will need to be made to obtain supplies abroad or for supplies to be carried by a companion.

Insulin used in the UK is now standardized to U100, but in some countries the availability of insulin may be limited in terms of type and strength. Individuals should elicit what insulin is available and what strengths it comes in, should insulin need to be obtained abroad. This is unlikely to be interchangeable with the individual's current method of delivery, so checking availability of pen devices/syringes is also necessary.

Travel to areas of high altitudes can cause the rubber bung in insulin pens to expand and contract, which can lead to air bubbles, and additional air shots may be necessary to remove these.

On arrival at the holiday destination insulin may be stored for up to 1month at room temperature. Storing in a fridge is not necessary, but avoidance of direct sun light is recommended.

Insulin tends to be absorbed more quickly in warmer climates, but more slowly in colder climates, and adjustments of insulin may be necessary to compensate for this.

Flights

During the flight it is recommended the individual chooses food from the airline menu, rather than ordering a special meal. Carrying additional snacks is recommended in case the airline food is unsuitable or in case of delays. The majority of airlines sell sugar-free drinks.

If the individual is crossing time zones or travelling for many hours, the dose and timing of insulin may need to be adjusted.

Time zones

General principles

- Check BG levels frequently.
- Maintain time on watch to local time. This will enable the individual to establish usual meal times and injections.
- If the time difference between departure and destination is less than 3h, continue usual routine.
- Flying east to west will add approximately 6h to the day. Therefore, additional insulin may be required. If on a basal bolus regime additional short- or rapid-acting insulin alongside a meal may be necessary. If on pre-mixed insulin, an additional injection may be needed or a dose of short- or rapid-acting insulin in addition to usual regime.
- Flying west to east shortens the day by approximately 6h. If on basal bolus regime, one less injection of short- or rapid-acting insulin may be required. If on pre-mixed insulin a reduction of dose should be sufficient.
- Establishing the usual regime as soon as possible is recommended on arrival at destination.

Holiday food

Enjoying local cuisine is all part of the social and cultural experience when travelling, but the food may contain more or less carbohydrate than is expected and fluctuations of BG levels may occur as a result. Individuals should be advised to avoid drinking tap water unless it has been declared safe to do so. Often individuals drink more alcohol than usual on holiday, which, associated with the potentially warmer climate, may increase the risk of hypoglycaemia (see 📖 p. 164).

If it is particularly hot, avoiding dehydration is essential. Individuals should be advised to increase their intake of low sugar drinks, including water.

Holiday illness

If illness develops during the holiday, individuals should be advised to maintain insulin and/or tablets, monitor BG levels frequently, and test urine for ketones, if appropriate.

Carbohydrate intake should be maintained in the form of regular sugary drinks, alternating with clear fluids to ensure fluid intake is maintained as much as possible. If the individual is vomiting persistently and is unable to keep any fluids down, they should be advised to seek medical help. If medical intervention is required, the individual should be advised to keep all receipts in order to claim against their holiday insurance on their return home.

Holiday activities

If the holiday is active, individuals will need to consider the effect of the activity on BG levels. If they are more active and in a warmer climate this may increase the risk of hypoglycaemia, so adjustments to insulin or additional snacks may be necessary. Alternatively, if the individual is less active and is eating more, additional insulin may be necessary.

Blood glucose monitoring

Many individuals see holidays as a good reason not to monitor BG, but for the majority of individuals, especially those with Type 2 diabetes on diet alone, or diet and oral hypoglycaemic agents, this may be possible, For those with Type 2 diabetes on insulin and Type 1 patients it is recommended they continue to monitor BG levels, as there are many aspects of holidays/travel that may influence diabetes control. To keep well and to ensure the diabetes does not interfere with the holiday, BG monitoring is recommended and it will be an essential tool during illness.

Further information

Diabetes UK ⊟ www.diabetes.org.uk
European Health Insurance Card ⊟ www.ehic.org.uk

Celebrations

Celebrations occur in a variety of formats – weddings, christenings, parties, etc. It is important that the individual with diabetes continues to enjoy celebrations as much as everybody else! With appropriate planning, celebrations can have minimal impact on diabetes control. For individuals with Type 2 diabetes on oral medications, the majority of medications can be taken at the usual times alongside food intake, if necessary, while for those individuals on insulin, both Types 1 and 2, an increase in insulin dose may be appropriate.

Stress/excitement

Often stress and excitement will lead to an increase in the release of counter-regulatory hormones, which will increase BG levels.

Injecting in public

A number of individuals are uncomfortable injecting in public, so when attending celebrations the individual may wish to consider where they may inject in privacy if necessary.

Monitoring blood glucose levels

Blood glucose levels may well be influenced by a number of factors relating to the celebration. The individual needs to decide if BG monitoring is necessary during the celebration. Blood glucose monitoring maybe beneficial before and after the event to establish how the diabetes control has been influenced and so that any changes to the individuals' regime can be implemented if necessary.

Alcohol

Often celebrations involve alcohol (see 📖 p. 284).

Food

Often the key issue surrounding celebrations is the timing, type, and quantity of food on offer. Where possible, establishing this before the event could be helpful. Carrying suitable snacks that could be eaten if the individual is uncomfortable with the menu on offer may also be beneficial. Often, during celebrations, people eat more than usual and accept that their BG levels will be higher. It is unlikely that individuals will suffer any consequences of this in the short term.

Avoiding hypoglycaemia

Avoiding hypoglycaemia is key to enjoying celebrations. If the individual is unclear when food will be served, carrying suitable snacks to bridge gaps between meals is helpful. Alcohol may also exacerbate hypoglycaemia (see 📖 p. 284). Carrying out their usual treatment for hypoglycaemia is essential.

Adjusting insulin

A number of people will adjust their insulin according to the event, potentially increasing it to take into account an increased food intake. Insulin should not be increased if it is anticipated that large quantities of alcohol will be consumed.

If the individual is not confident adjusting insulin doses, there may need to be a level of acceptance that the BG control may be influenced on the day/evening of the celebration. This will not influence their long-term outcomes with diabetes.

Alcohol

The current recommendations for safe limits of alcohol are:
- **For men:** 21units/week or 3units/day.
- **For women:** 14units/week or 2units/day.

It is recommended that individuals have 2 or 3 alcohol-free days per week.

Examples of 1unit of alcohol
- ½pint ordinary beer or lager.
- Small glass of wine.
- Single measure of spirit.

Special considerations in diabetes
- Alcohol is high in calories and can contribute to weight gain, high bp, and hyperlipidaemia. For the individual with Type 2 diabetes, which in most cases require the individual to lose weight, reducing alcohol consumption may facilitate weight loss.
- Low-sugar beers and lagers are not recommended as the alcohol content tends to be higher, and in low alcohol beers/lagers the glucose content is higher. Therefore, 'ordinary' beers and lagers are recommended.
- If required, spirits should be mixed with sugar-free mixers.

Alcohol and hypoglycaemia

Alcohol is metabolized in the liver. This reduces the ability of the liver to enable gluconeogenesis and, therefore, increases the risk of hypoglycaemia. This may occur several hours after alcohol has been consumed. It is recommended that individuals with diabetes do not consume alcohol on an empty stomach, ensuring they have a meal or snack before drinking and, if possible, performing a BG test before bed to establish if further snacking is required is recommended.

Cultural considerations

Diabetes care is being provided in a rapidly changing environment. The cultural mix of the UK population may present challenges for care providers and individuals with diabetes. Culture is defined as a way of life shared by members of society – it incorporates learned beliefs, values, behaviours, and traditions that are the norm for a group of people who are unified by race, ethnicity, language, nationality, or religion.

Health care professionals (HCPs) must ensure they have sufficient knowledge to meet the demands of various cultures and beliefs. The environment that the HCP works within will influence the knowledge and skills necessary for managing specific groups.

Type 2 diabetes prevalence is higher and occurs in the younger age groups of African/Caribbean and Asian backgrounds and development of micro- and macrovascular complications is higher in ethnic communities.

Factors to be considered when caring for cultural differences and diabetes

Dietary habits

- Eating habits may vary widely between ethnic groups, and types and timings of meals can be different.
- Sweet foods are often included as part of celebrations and festivities, and many individuals would not refuse these sweets foods.
- Fasting is common among some cultures.
- Obesity may be viewed as a sign of wealth and prosperity.
- Certain foods, including alcohol, may be prohibited and it may be considered offensive to ask a member of the Muslim community if they drink alcohol.
- A full dietary assessment is helpful in establishing types and timings of meals, and how these may differ during festivities and celebrations.

Ramadan

This is the holy month for Muslims, during which they fast from dawn till sunset. It is obligatory for all healthy adult Muslims with the exception of the elderly, children under 12, pregnant and breast feeding women, and those who are considered sick. People with diabetes can be exempt from fasting, although many choose not to. If this is the case, the following will need consideration:

- Only 2 meals are typically eaten per day, sunrise and sunset, and these meals tend to be high in sweet foods.
- Hypoglycaemia risk is higher for those on insulin and sulphonylureas.
- To avoid hypoglycaemia, timings of insulin and sulphonylureas may need to change.

Medications

Herbal medications may be taken alongside traditional diabetes treatment, some of which may influence diabetes control. Therefore, it is important to establish if and what individuals may be taking.

Some cultures will not accept animal insulin. In the Muslim and Jewish cultures, where pork or its products are forbidden, pork insulin will not be used. Similarly, Sikhs would not consider using beef insulin. This is unlikely to present any problems as insulins today are genetically manufactured, although individuals from these cultures may wish to establish the origin of insulin.

Provision of care

Language barriers remain the most challenging aspect of providing diabetes care to culturally diverse groups. Interpreters may be necessary and, where possible, qualified interpreters are recommended. Unless the HCP can speak the language, it is difficult to know how the information is being translated.

Establishing health care beliefs is essential, and the HCP should establish, as far as possible, the cultural differences and how these may influence dietary habits, taking medications, and being engaged in diabetes care.

Consultations and examinations

The HCP also needs to establish custom and practice with regard to consultations and examinations. Women from some cultures may need to be examined by a lady doctor and/or nurse. Removal of clothing may not be acceptable in some cultures and examining feet may be problematic.

Further information

A wide range of leaflets are provided in consideration of cultural differences and in various languages from: 🖳 www.diabetes.org.uk.

Smoking

There is a growing body of evidence to suggest that smoking is an independent risk factor for diabetes as it increases insulin resistance. In smokers insulin resistance has been shown to be markedly aggravated in Type 2 diabetes (Will, 2001). Therefore, there is an increased risk of developing Type 2 diabetes in the smoking population.

For people with established diabetes, smoking aggravates the risk of serious disease and premature death. The increased risk of heart disease already increases the risk of premature death in Type 2 diabetes, smoking increases this risk. There is also an association with increased risk of cardiovascular death. A large prospective study demonstrated that the relative risks for mortality were:

• 1.31 for past smokers.
• 1.43 for current smokers who smoked up to 14 cigarettes per day.
• 1.64 for current smokers who smoked 15–34 cigarettes per day.
• 2.19 for current smokers who smoked 35 plus cigarettes per day (Al-Delaimy, 2001).

Smoking is associated with multiple complications of diabetes, including an increased risk of nephropathy. Albuminuria rates are increased in Types 1 and 2 diabetes, and it has also been demonstrated that the incidence of neuropathy is higher in smokers for both types of diabetes.

Smoking cessation

There is overwhelming evidence that stopping smoking reduces the risk of cardio- and cerebrovascular disease, lung disease, and cancer. As diabetes increases the risk of cardio- and cerebrovascular disease, it follows that stopping smoking will reduce the risks of long-term complications and diabetes. Unfortunately, the evidence is largely circumstantial, as few studies have evaluated smoking cessation specifically in diabetes.

Although in a large USA study, stopping smoking was associated with a reduction in risk of premature death, women with Type 2 diabetes who had stopped smoking for 10 years or more had a mortality risk comparable with women with Type 2 diabetes who had never smoked

There are many barriers to smoking cessation – one frequently cited is the fear of weight gain. This is particularly relevant in diabetes as weight gain often will influence BG control, as insulin resistance increases with the associated weight gain. This may necessitate an increase in diabetes therapy insulin and/ or oral hypoglycaemic agents.

Further information

Al-Delaimy WK, Willett WC, Manson JE, et al. (2001) Smoking and mortality among women with Type 2 diabetes: the nurses' health study cohort. *Diabet Care* **12**, 2043–8.

Will JC. (2001) Cigarette smoking and diabetes: evidence of a positive association form a large prospective cohort study. *Int J Epidemiol* **30**, 554–5.

For help on stopping smoking refer patients to QUIT: ⌨ www.quit.org.uk, or ⌨ www.gosmoke-free.co.uk.

Recreational drugs

Recreational drugs not only carry risks associated with general health, they carry increased risks for people with diabetes. The effects will be variable depending on what drug is being used, the quantity, and frequency.

Recreational drugs affect individuals in varying ways and all will affect the individual's behaviour, and the ability to self-manage their diabetes and to recognize hypoglycaemia, and increase the risk for diabetic ketoacidosis.

Recreational drugs can be divided broadly into 3 main categories.

Stimulants ('Uppers')

This category includes speed, ecstasy, and cocaine. These drugs tend to increase heart rate, and are often taken to increase energy. Used regularly, stimulants cause confusion, mood swings, and aggression. The higher rate of metabolism experienced can lead to dehydration. Any stimulant that changes the rate of metabolism will affect BG levels. If vomiting occurs, associated with the potential dehydration, this class of drug exacerbates the potential for diabetic ketoacidosis to increase.

Depressants ('Downers')

Including alcohol and heroin, alcohol is the most commonly used in this group. Excessive alcohol can lead to poor judgement, slowed reflexes, and potential collapse. Vomiting after too much alcohol is common and this can influence diabetes control, especially if the vomiting is prolonged. The effects of alcohol can sometimes mask the symptoms of hypoglycaemia or the individual may be viewed as hypoglycaemic when, in actual fact, they are drunk! (see 📖 Hypoglycaemia: causes, p. 164).

Heroin is an opiate. It slows the brain's reactions, including individuals' perceptions and the way they think. It is highly addictive, causing strong physical and psychological dependence. It can reduce appetite and affect the ability to recognize hypos and it affects motivation. Self-managing diabetes may be extremely difficult if an individual uses heroin.

Hallucinogenic

Includes cannabis and acid solvents. Cannabis is the most commonly used illegal drug. Hallucinogenic drugs tend to:
- Change the individuals' perceptions of their immediate environment. Often a sense of time is lost, and managing eating and insulin regimes can therefore be difficult. Missing insulin frequently could lead to diabetic ketoacidosis.
- Hallucinogenic drugs can also make individuals feel panicky and light headed.
- As they affect short-term memory there is an increased risk of forgetting to take medications or insulin.
- Often appetite is increased, frequently uncontrolled, and this is likely to increase BG levels.

Useful websites

Alcohol Concern 🖳 www.alcoholconcern.org.uk
Action on Smoking and Health 🖳 www.ash.org.uk
Drug Scope 🖳 www.drugscope.org.uk

Chapter 13

Managing investigations and procedures

Fluids only

Before undergoing surgery or an investigative procedure people with diabetes may need to fast and perhaps restrict themselves to fluid-only intake. There will be specific, written, pre- and peri-operative guidelines for the area in which you work, although there may be minor variations in these guidelines from place to place. It is imperative that you adhere to the guidelines specific to your hospital, otherwise, in the event of a problem, your employer may not accept vicarious liability for your actions.

Three main areas to assess for people with diabetes are:
• Long-term complications of diabetes: these will complicate the peri-operative and recovery management. Check urea and electrolytes (see 📖 Chapter 9, pp. 179–218).
• Glucose control (HbA1C) prior to admission, or any recent hypo or hyperglycaemia
  • recent repeated hypoglycaemia will lower the threshold at which the patient is aware of hypo and may lead to unstable BG levels;
  • pre-operative hyperglycaemia will impair healing and, therefore, recovery.

Ensure blood glucose (BG) is carefully controlled during and following surgery or the procedure.

Nil by mouth

Where possible, for any operation or procedure, it is easier if the person with diabetes is placed on the theatre list early in the morning.

Minor surgery, endoscopy, or investigations

For people with Type 2 diabetes on oral hypoglycaemics and those managed on diet alone

Pre-operatively

- Omit any hypoglycaemic therapy on the day of surgery.
- Avoid glucose infusions.
- Check BG regularly.
- Restart oral medication with the first meal following the procedure. For patients with renal impairment following surgery, metformin may be withheld until kidney function is resumed, as there is an association between metforim and lactic acidosis.
- Metformin should be stopped prior to procedures involving the use of iodine containing X-ray contrast medium, e.g. angiography (please refer to local guidelines).

For all people who use insulin pre-operatively

- Check pre-operative BG control is optimized (HbA1C preferably in target range).
- Consider changes in insulin regimen peri-operatively, e.g. twice daily to multiple injections.
- For those on multiple injection therapy, consider continuing with their usual long-acting basal insulin.
- On the morning of the operation:
  - check BG and recheck hourly pre-, intra-, and post operatively.
  - commence an iv infusion of glucose and insulin (unless anaesthetist requests otherwise);
  - ensure the patient's normal doses of rapid-acting or mixed insulins are **omitted**.

For all people who use insulin post-operatively

- When patient is eating normally resume subcutaneous (sc) insulin.
- Continue the iv insulin until the sc has begun to be absorbed.
- Maintain good BG control.

Major surgery

All patients will require iv insulin following fasting.

Day case surgery for people on insulin therapy

- Aim for the patient to be first on the list.
- For those on a multiple injection regime, continue the usual long-acting basal insulin the evening prior to the procedure (consider a 10–20% reduction).
- For those on bd insulin, continue the usual evening insulin (consider a 10–20% reduction).
- Fast from midnight and **omit** the morning insulin.
- Check BG regularly before and after the procedure.
- Resume the usual insulin regime and diet after the procedure.
- If a bd insulin regimen is restarted at lunchtime, it is recommended that half of the normal 'breakfast' insulin dose should be given with lunch.

The above applies if rapid recovery is expected, i.e. the patient is expected to be eating within 2h of the procedure. If the patient is unable to tolerate diet or the BG is high (perhaps >14mmol/l), follow the protocols relevant to your place of work.

Laser treatment for macular oedema or proliferate retinopathy

(see 📖 Retinopathy: diabetic eye disease, p. 210)

Treatment and follow-up appointments will normally be offered as an out-patient at the local hospital's Ophthalmology Department (the eye clinic) and may be carried out over several appointments.

It is important to remind patients that pupil dilating drops are instilled into both their eyes before a fundoscopy examination prior to the laser treatment and they should:
• Not drive themselves home.
• Wear dark glasses home.

Anaesthetic drops are administered to the eye undergoing the laser treatment and a special lens inserted for the duration of the procedure. This helps to keep the eye lids fully open and to focus the rays from the laser onto the retina.

Patients may be reassured that they will get used to the dazzling brightness during their laser treatment and that the treatment is normally painless, but some minor discomfort may be experienced.

Their sight will be affected for a few hours following the laser, but hopefully will be back to normal by the next day, although some patients complain of blurred vision for 2–3 days post-treatment. Any residual discomfort, especially if they have had a lot of treatment sessions, may be treated with paracetamol or aspirin.

Considerations for in-patient care

Standard 8 of the National Service Framework (NSF) for Diabetes (2001) states that:

> All children, young people, and adults with diabetes admitted to hospital, for whatever reason, will receive effective care of their diabetes. Wherever possible they will continue to be involved in decisions concerning the management of their diabetes. (p. 33)

This raises the following considerations:
- Adequate staff training to enable them confidently and knowledgeably to deliver care to people with diabetes.
- Employment of specialist nurses to oversee the management of the care administered to people with diabetes, whilst they are in-patients.
- Vigilance regarding the appropriate timing of meals, snacks, and medication.
- The provision of protocols or guidelines regarding:
  - self-testing and self-administration of insulin, whilst an in-patient
  - involvement regarding decisions concerning their diabetes care
  - provision and availability of healthier food and snack options
  - provision of and access to ethnic minority and religious observance food choices
  - monitoring and measurement of BG control
  - iv infusion regimens
  - wound management
  - timing of investigations and procedures
  - provision of clear information detailing what to expect during their stay in hospital and following their discharge home.

Adapted from *NSF for diabetes* (2001).

Further information

DoH (2001) *National Service Framework for Diabetes: standards.* HMSO, London.

Chapter 14

Organization of care

National agenda for managing patients with long-term conditions

The Department of Health (DoH) estimates that there are 15.4 million people with a long-term condition (LTC) in England. It has been essential that strategies that maximize the efficacy and efficiency of their care should be developed. These strategies fundamentally apply to the delivery of care for people with diabetes who number 1,962,000 of those with a LTC (QOF). The prevalence of LTCs in the population is age-related, with 3 in every 5 people aged over 60 years identified as being treated for a LTC.

The modernization agenda

To describe the Government's agenda of modernization, and the delivery of evidence-based and co-ordinated care, they have developed a web site that outlines their non-clinical guidelines to enable holistic and patient-centred individualized care delivery (🖳 http://www.dh.gov.uk/en/Healthcare/Longterm conditions/index.htm)

The modernization agenda lists 5 high-level outcomes for care delivery, all of which are pertinent for caring for people with diabetes. They are:
• People have improved quality of life, health, and wellbeing, and are enabled to be more independent.
• People are supported, self-care is enabled, and patients have an active involvement in decisions about their care and support.
• People have choice and control over their care and support so that services are built around their needs.
• People can design their care around health and social care services, which are integrated, flexible, proactive, and responsive to individual needs.
• People are offered health and social care services, which are high quality, efficient, and sustainable.

The DoH document *Long term conditions compendium of information: adding life to years and years to life* (2008) sets further objectives.

Better health and well-being for all
Helping people to stay:
• Healthy and well.
• Empowering people to live independently.
• Tackling health inequalities.

Better care for all
The best possible health and social care, offering safe and effective services, when and where people need help, and empowering people to make choices.

Better value for all
- Affordable.
- Efficient.
- Sustainable services.
- Contributing to the wider economy and the nation.

The indicators set to measure the success of these initiatives are:
- Increased patient satisfaction with the health and support they receive.
- Their ability to be in control of their condition.
- A reduction in the use of emergency bed days.

These will be achieved through changes to the infrastructure of community resources dividing care delivery between primary, secondary, and community care services.

Further information

Department of Health (2008) *Long term conditions compendium of information: adding life to years and years to life*. DoH, London. Available at: http://www.dh.gov.uk/en/Healthcare/Longtermconditions/index.htm (accessed 16 April 2009)

Department of Health (2008). *Quality and Outcomes Framework 2006/07*. HMSO: London.

Structure of care delivery organizations: primary care

Structure

In the English NHS model, this is the part of the health service that delivers care through:

- Family doctors (GPs).
- Community and practice nurses.
- Community therapists (such as physiotherapists and occupational therapists)
- Community pharmacists.
- Optometrists.
- Dentists.
- Midwives.

Primary Care Trusts (PCTs) are free-standing organizations with their own boards, staff members, and budgets, and are monitored by their local Strategic Health Authority (SHA). They commission and provide care directly. Commissioning of care is being extended in two ways: first, to practice-based commissioning (PBC) where practices and other health care professionals (HCPs) are encouraged to take part in commissioning local services. Secondly, PCTs and local authorities are to join at a strategic level – forming Local Strategic Partnerships and develop a health and social care environment network which includes:

- Joint commissioning posts.
- Pooled budgets.
- Joint public health departments.
- Joint strategic needs assessment.
- Liaison with the 'third sector' (employment and housing).
- The use of local involvement networks.
- Partnership working and collaboration at all levels:
  - PCTs;
  - GP practices;
  - primary and secondary care;
  - the acute sector.
- Integrated working between health and social care involving multidisciplinary teams creating a more holistic approach for service provision based around the needs of individuals.

Primary care will be provided with decision support tools and clinical information systems (NPfIT), which will provide the tools to optimize the gathering of good information necessary to underpin:

- Strategic needs assessment.
- Commissioning.
- Risk stratification.
- Early and appropriate prevention and targeting interventions.

These new IT systems will include quality and outcome frameworks to drive and incentivize improvements.

Decision support software will be developed using:
- National Strategic Frameworks.
- National Institute for Health and Clinical Excellence (NICE) guidance.
- Evidence-based practice (EBP).

Structure of care delivery organizations: secondary care

This part of English NHS service provision comprises the acute hospitals, which are in the process of being reconfigured as part of the government initiative aimed at enhancing the range of NHS acute hospital provision near to patient's homes.

Other new proposals within this sector include:
- Booked admissions.
- Expanding day surgery provision.
- Pathology and radiology modernization.
- NHS Foundation Trusts.

Within the hospitals, which make up the secondary care provision, are the **emergency care services.** In 2001, a 10-year strategy, *Reforming Emergency Care*, was published. This drove changes in emergency care, and gave priority to staff and patients in emergency care settings. This unplanned care is considered under the following headings:
- Ambulance provision and paramedics.
- Critical care.
- Minor illness and injury.

In addition **NHS Direct** is a national telephone service, which offers advice, given by trained nurses, directly to the patient. This service is commissioned by local PCTs and is delivered as two distinct services:
- **Nationally-directed services:** covering the national core 0845 4647 service.
- **NHS DirectOnline** and Digital TV services.

Further information

Department of Health guidelines. *Configuring hospitals.* ⌨ http://www.dh.gov.uk/en/Healthcare/Secondarycare/Configuringhospitals/index.htm

Structure of care delivery organizations: intermediate and integrated care

Intermediate care

Positioned to interface between the primary and secondary care systems are the **Intermediate Care Teams**. In 2001, Health Authorities, Primary Care Groups/Trusts, NHS Trusts, and councils were encouraged to better integrate social and health care (DoH, 2001). One intention was the reduction of delayed discharges and since 2004 there has been a financial disincentive for local authorities who have not provided supporting community care arrangements.

Integrated care

Pilot programmes, empowering clinicians to work closely with their partners, including patients, to lead the testing of new models of integration are based on one or more GP registered list populations and will run for 2 years (DoH, 2008).

Further information

Department of Health (2001) *Health Service Circular (HSC) 2001/001 Intermediate care.* HMSO, London.

Department of Health (2008) *Integrated care pilot programme – prospectus for potential pilots,* HMSO, London.

Multi-professional, multi-disciplinary, and integrated diabetes care delivery

The National Service Frameworks (NSF) for Diabetes, standards and delivery strategy, envisaged care that is patient focused and delivered in line with the principles laid out in the *NHS Plan* and *The Expert Patient*. Because diabetes care involves multiprofessional, multidisciplinary, and integrated care delivery, crossing the artificial boundaries between primary and secondary care, it exemplifies the notion of a seamless service of shared care, shared between the professionals whatever their discipline and wherever they work, and shared with the patient.

The NSF for Diabetes (standards) sets out the facets of care delivery as:
• Prevention.
• Diagnosis.
• Initial care.
• Continuing care.

The NHS and partner agencies are tasked with reviewing locality provision of diabetes services to identify any deficiencies and to audit the protocols set out in the NSF across each of these 4 areas, in both primary and secondary care.

An example of this cross-sector approach may be found in Standard 7 of the NSF for diabetes (DoH, 2001a), which refers to the Management of Diabetic Emergencies. The interventions outlined range from the provision of 'rapid and effective treatment of diabetic emergencies by appropriately trained health care professionals'. These emergencies include diabetic ketoacidosis (DKA) (see 📖 p. 172) and hyperosmolar non-ketotic syndrome (HONK) (sometimes called hyperosmolar coma, 📖 p. 174), both of which are life-threatening and usually treated in the secondary sector by personnel such as:
• Paramedics.
• Ambulance personnel.
• GPs.
• Accident and emergency staff.
• Intensive or dependency care staff.

However, it often necessitates the recognition and initial management of these emergencies by those in primary care settings such as:
• Community nursing.
• Dental practices.
• Practice nurse clinics.
• Podiatry.
• Minor injury and accident departments.
• Community hospitals.
• Respite care placements.

Further information

Department of Health (2000) *NHS Plan*. HMSO, London.

Department of Health (2001a) *National Service Framework for Diabetes*, Standards. HMSO, London.

Department of Health (2001b) *The Expert Patient: a new approach to chronic disease management in the 21st century*. HMSO, London.

NHS Modernisation Agency (2005) *Case management competences framework for the care of people with long term conditions*. Available at: www.dh.gov.uk/en/Publicationsandstatistics/Publications/PublicationspolicyandGuidance/DH_4118101 (accessed 16 April 2009).

Department of Health (2005) *Supporting people with long term conditions: Liberating the talents of nurses who care for people with long term conditions*. Available at: www.dh.gov.uk/en/Publicationsandstatistics/Publications/PublicationsPolicyandGuidance/DH_4102469 (accessed 16 April 2009).

Department of Health (2006) *Caring for people with long term conditions: an education framework for community matrons and case managers*. Available at: www.dh.gov.uk/en/Publicationsandstatistics/Publications/PublicationsPolicyandGuidance/DH_4133997 (accessed 16 April 2009).

Department of Health (2006) *How a community matron can help you with your long term condition*. Available at: www.dh.gov.uk/en/Publicationsandstatistics/Publications/PublicationsPolicyandGuidance/DH_4133998 (accessed 16 April 2009).

Residential care

The care delivered to people who reside in care homes is regulated under the Care Standards Act (DoH, 2000). People with diabetes should receive these minimal standards of clinical care:

- **Standard 1:** each adult resident in a care home will be screened annually for diabetes.
- **Standard 2:** each resident with diabetes will have their diabetes care documented in their care plan.
- **Standard 3:** each resident will have an annual review of their diabetes in the most appropriate setting.
- **Standard 4:** each care home will have a named member of staff, trained in the care of people with diabetes. This training will cover such areas as:
  - types of diabetes;
  - importance of good BG control, monitoring, and interpretation of results;
  - quality of life and risk management issues in diabetes care;
  - cultural and ethical issues involved in diabetes care;
  - avoidance and management of hypoglycaemia;
  - screening for complications, e.g. foot care, eye disease, and cardiovascular disease;
  - principles of the diabetic diet;
  - care in intercurrent illness;
  - their role in care plan development, management, and the annual review process;
  - the role of Diabetes UK and voluntary bodies.

When a resident with diabetes does not wish to receive this care, it should be documented in their care record and their General Practitioner informed (see also 📖 Care home residency, p. 262).

Further information

Department of Health (2001) *The Care Homes for Older People National Minimum Standards.* HMSO, London.

Diabetes UK (2003) *What diabetes care to expect.* Diabetes UK, London.

National Institute for Clinical Excellence (2002) *Management of Type 2 diabetes.* NICE, London. Available at: 🖥 www.nice.org.uk (accessed 16 April 2009).

National Institute for Clinical Excellence (2004) *Type 1 diabetes: diagnosis and management of type 1 diabetes in children and young people.* NICE, London. Available at: 🖥 www.nice.org.uk (accessed 16 April 2009).

National Service Framework for Diabetes: Standards (2001). Available at: 🖥 www.dh.gov.uk/en/ Healthcare/NationalServiceFrameworks/Diabetes/index.htm (accessed 16 April 2009).

National Service Framework for Older People (2001). Available at: 🖥 www.dh.gov.uk/en/ SocialCare/Deliveringadultsocialcare/Olderpeople/OlderpeopleNSFstandards/index.htm (accessed 16 April 2009).

Philosophy of care

In order to direct the delivery of care for people with diabetes it is important that every team undertaking this work spend some time reflecting upon the ways in which they work.

The NSF for care of people with diabetes and the NICE guidelines have empowerment of patients, self-care, and management of the condition at their heart. In order for patients to have the skills, knowledge, and understanding to optimize their clinical parameters and wellbeing, they require timely and appropriate educational input.

For example, the NHS Type 1 educational philosophy has been encapsulated in the following points.

The person with diabetes has the right to expect the following from their health care professional:
- The development of an open, honest, and non-hierarchical relationship with the person with diabetes.
- An approach that treats the person as an individual, is respectful of their health beliefs, and is supportive, consistent, and non-judgemental.
- An opportunity to identify and review the person's needs, concerns, and goals.
- The provision of up-to-date, accurate, and consistent information about diabetes, treatment options, and local services (e.g. education programmes) available, in order to address their needs and concerns, and help meet their goals.

The health care professional will achieve this by:
- Engaging with the person with diabetes and gaining their trust.
- Identifying and exploring their current health beliefs and factors that motivate current self-care behaviours.
- Helping the person to explore and understand the risks and benefits of their current situation/management choice, and of any alternative options.
- Providing appropriate information to support decision-making.
- Providing or providing access to knowledge and skills needed to achieve self-care behaviour appropriate to each decision.

New developments

Treatments: 1

Implications of stem cell legislatory changes

In May 2008 an attempt to ban the experimentation on hybrid embryos was defeated in the House of Commons. The Human Fertilization and Embryology Bill could change the law on embryo research for the first time in 20 years, allowing regulated research using hybrid (admix) embryos. A hybrid is formed when nuclei of human embryonic cells are inserted into 'empty' animal eggs. It is planned that the resultant embryos will be allowed to develop for 14 days and stem cells will then be harvested. It is hoped that research using these cells could lead to greater knowledge regarding Type 1 diabetes and other serious debilitating conditions.

Research developments in stem cell production

Teams from the Universities of Sheffield and Manchester have been able to genetically modify stem cells to produce the protein PAX4 or 'transcription factor'. It was found that PAX4 encouraged a large number (about 20%) of stem cells to become pancreatic beta cells, which have the potential to produce insulin when transplanted into the body. Dr Karen Cosgrove, a research scientist supported on this project by the Juvenile Diabetes Research Forum (JDRF) told their open meeting in April 2008 that usually less than 1% of stem cells develop to be insulin producing pancreatic cells.

The Xcell-centre diabetes mellitus treatment

Adult stem cell therapy, costing between 6000 and 9000 euros per treatment, has been piloted on 23 people with Type 1 and Type 2 diabetes. Here stem cells, collected from the patient's iliac crest bone marrow, are implanted back into their body several days later. These cells have the potential to develop into pancreatic beta cells. The research published following a 6 month study by X-cell-centre.com showed that 10 of the 23 patients treated had reduced their insulin/oral hypoglycaemic medication requirements by between 20 and 50% without a worsening of their HbA1c levels.

Islet transplants carried out by the NHS

Diabetes UK Research Matters magazine reported in their Spring 2008 issue that the Department of Health (DoH) had announced a pledge to spend £2.34 million in islet transplantation in 2008, rising to £7.32 million per year. They noted the dangers inherent in the use of immunosuppressant drugs that has led the DoH to restrict transplants to patients who experience severe recurrent hypoglycaemia or have had a kidney transplant. They note that transplantation, which is still an experimental procedure, will take place at:

- Oxford Radcliffe Hospitals NHS Foundation Trust.
- Royal Free Hospital and King's College Hospital, London.
- Newcastle-upon-Tyne Hospitals NHS Trust.
- North Bristol NHS Trust.
- Central Manchester and Manchester Children's NHS Trust.

NICE guidelines (October 2003) split the procedures into two – allogeneic pancreatic islet cell transplantation for Type 1 diabetes and autologous pancreatic islet cell transplantation for improved glycaemic control after pancreatectomy.

Incretin hormone glucagon-like peptide-1 (GLP1) therapy or dipeptidyl peptidase IV inhibitors

GLP1s are currently in clinical development for the treatment of Type 2 diabetes and show hopeful results in the improvement of glucose homeostasis (Combettes, 2006).

In people with Type 2 diabetes, the GLP1 response is significantly reduced or absent. The circulating half life of GLP1 is short due to the rapid degradation by the enzyme dipeptidyl peptidase (DPP-IV).

The principle action of GLP1 is to:

- Increase endogenous insulin secretion in response to BG levels.
- Reduce hepatic gluconeogenesis.
- Delay gastric emptying.
- Increase satiety.

Incretin-based therapies seek either to replace deficient levels of GLP1, e.g. exenatide, or to prevent the degradation of GLP1 by DPP-IV using DPP-IV inhibitors, e.g. sitagliptin.

Further information

Department of Health ▫ www.dh.gov.uk
NICE ▫ www.nice.org.uk
Diabetes UK Research Matters ▫ www.diabetes.org.uk/Research/Publications/Research_matters
Combettes, MMJ (2006) GLP-1 and type 2 diabetes: physiology and new clinical advances.
   Curr Opin Pharmacol **6**, 598–605.

Treatments: 2

New genetic findings for people with Type 2 diabetes

16 areas on the human genome have been implicated in the development of Type 2 diabetes. People with a particular version of *CAPN10* are more likely to develop Type 2 diabetes than those without that version. The research teams at St Bartholomew's and the London School of Medicine and Dentistry, led by Dr Mark Turner, have shown that the protein called Calpain-10, produced by *CAPN10* gene, is responsible for enabling the release of intracellular insulin into the blood stream. They have shown that increasing the activity of the gene increases the insulin secretion. This is facilitated as the protein rearranges the intracellular transport system moving the insulin pockets to the cells surface from where insulin is released into the blood stream.

There is, therefore, a potential that new drug developments may be able to activate existing *CAPN10* and these could be used to treat people with the faulty version of the gene. Alternatively, it may be possible to replace the faulty *CAPN10* with a correct genetic sequence.

New approach to treating Type 2 diabetes

A 3-year project led by Professor O'Harte at the University of Ulster has enabled a modified version of the gut hormone GIP to be developed. GIP is post-prandially secreted from intestinal cells and is capable of lowering BG concentrations. It is known to stimulate both insulin secretion and pancreatic beta-cell growth, but is degraded by DPP-IV, an enzyme circulating in the blood. GIP is also excreted through the kidneys.

Mice, with Type 2 diabetes, given a modified version of GIP, had improved glycaemic control without increased hypoglycaemia. This is because GIP is only active in the presence of glucose. The modifications made to GIP prolonged its duration of action and the most promising versions of GIP will be taken forward to clinical trials (Diabetes UK, 2008).

Possible drug for eye condition

Clinical trials carried out by researchers at Johns Hopkins University in Baltimore, Maryland, showed that a drug called ranibizumab is effective against diabetic macular oedema, a major complication that often leads to vision loss. Ranibizumab, an existing drug with a licence for a different application, works by blocking the effects of a protein called VEGF, which causes leakage in the eye's tiny blood vessels. NICE guidelines for the drugs were released in the summer of 2008.

Further information

Diabetes UK (2008) *Research Matters*, Spring, **7**. Available at: ▣ www.diabetes.org.uk

Discoveries

Possible causes of circulatory problems in people with Type 2 diabetes

Research funded by the British Heart Foundation has enabled University of Bristol researchers to identify a protein receptor p75NTR, which is found in the cells of mice with diabetes. p75NTR seems to:
- Inhibit the growth of new blood vessels.
- Reduce blood vessel function.
- Lead to poor circulation.
- Slow wound healing.

Suppressing the gene that produces p75NTR improves the circulation in mice with Type 2 diabetes. Healthy cells that heal quickly do not have p75NTR and if the receptor is put into them they become dysfunctional. These findings have implications for people with diabetes who, at present, undergo limb amputation because of poor circulation.

Approaches to care

Eating disorders

Dr Tierney, a lead researcher on a Diabetes UK project at the University of Manchester has found that health professionals, including doctors and nurses, do not routinely assess people with Type 1 diabetes for eating disorders.

Research has been carried that demonstrates the pressure on young people to be extremely slim, and to try to attain the impossible body shapes depicted in magazines and by the media (Nielsen, 2002). It has been noted that some people with Type 1 diabetes deliberately allow their BG levels to run high, as this enables them to remain slim. It is noted that adults with Type 1 diabetes may have bulimia nervosa, anorexia nervosa, and/or use insulin dose manipulation.

NICE guidelines (2004) state:

> **1.4.3.1** Diabetes care teams should be aware that children and young people with Type 1 diabetes, in particular young women, have an increased risk of eating disorders.
>
> **1.4.3.2** Diabetes care teams should be aware that children and young people with Type 1 diabetes who have eating disorders may have associated problems of persistent hyperglycaemia, recurrent hypoglycaemia and/ or symptoms associated with gastric paresis.
>
> **1.4.3.3** Children and young people with Type 1 diabetes in whom eating disorders are identified by their diabetes care team should be offered joint management involving their diabetes care.

It is essential that those offering care to people with Type 1 diabetes do so sensitively, and are aware of the possibility, implications and consequences of eating disorders, and the availability of support regarding safe BG levels, nutritional advice, and treatment for these patients.

Psychological support for adults with diabetes

Research from Leeds General Infirmary, the Institute of Psychiatry and Diabetes UK, focused on the nature and availability of psychological services for adults with diabetes in the UK. A study of 267 centres treating people with diabetes showed 64% did not comply with national standards, such as the NSFs or guidelines, although they recognized the importance of these issues.

This raises huge implications for practice in establishing and running facilities where none exist at the moment. There is also the need to train more health care professionals who are able to treat and support adults with diabetes requiring psychological support in the UK.

Further information

NICE (2004) *Type 1 diabetes: diagnosis and management of Type 1 diabetes in children, young people and adults*, Clinical guideline 15. NICE, London. Available at: 🖳 www.nice.org.uk

Nielsen S. (2002) Eating disorders in females with Type 1 diabetes: an update of a meta-analysis. *Eur Eating Disord Rev* **10**, 241–54.

Chapter 16

Policy

Diabetes policy: England

National Service Framework for Diabetes

Following consultation with doctors, nurses, NHS executives, voluntary bodies such as Diabetes UK, and people with diabetes, the Department of Health (DoH) issued the *National Service Framework (NSF) for Diabetes, Standards* policy document. In his foreword, Alan Millburn, the then Secretary of State for Health, avowed it was the intention of the NSF to 'make best practice the norm' (DoH 2001 *NSF for Diabetes Standards*, p. 2).

The standards framework was followed 1year later by the *NSF for Diabetes Delivery Strategy* and in August 2002 the *National Service Frameworks: a practical aid to implementation in primary care.*

The following 12 Standards were listed in the NSF:
- **Standard 1:** Prevention of Type 2 diabetes.
- **Standard 2**: Identification of people with diabetes.
- **Standard 3:** Empowering people with diabetes.
- **Standard 4:** Clinical care of adults with diabetes.
- **Standards 5 and 6:** Clinical care of children and young people with diabetes.
- **Standard 7:** Management of diabetic emergencies.
- **Standard 8:** Care of people with diabetes during admission to hospital.
- **Standard 9:** Diabetes and pregnancy.
- **Standards 10,11, and 12:** Detection and management of long term conditions.

DoH publications in 2004

Management of medicines: a resource to support implementation of the wider aspects of medicines management for the NSF for diabetes, renal and long-term conditions. Provides practical examples of innovative practice in medicines management techniques.

DoH publications in 2006

- **A guide to commissioning diabetes services, the *Diabetes Commissioning Toolkit* :** A best practice guide providing practical advice for all commissioners of diabetes services downloadable as a PDF from: 🖳 www.dh.gov.uk/en/Publicationsandstatistics/Publications/PublicationsPolicyAndGuidance/DH_4140284
- *Turning the corner: improving diabetes care* was published by the DoH, and outlines improvements and challenges to the service in the first 3 years following publication of the NSF.
- *Care planning in diabetes: report from the joint DoH and Diabetes UK Care and planning working group:* this report provides advice regarding care planning linking with standard 3 of the NSF.

DoH publications in 2007

- *Working together for better diabetes care:* the National Director for Diabetes sets out strategies to facilitate care delivery by a team approach.
- *The way ahead – the local challenge improving diabetes services:* report highlighting the service developments over the first 4 years since the NSF.
- *Making every young person with diabetes matter:* report indicating current problems providing guidance and making recommendations in areas, including commissioning, organization of care, provision of services, and workforce planning.

Guidance on the use of educational models for diabetes education is available from NICE HTA No 60.

Reference

Department of Health (2001) *National Service Framework for Diabetes: Standards.* HMSO, London.

Diabetes policy: Scotland

In 2001 the Scottish Intercollegiate Guidelines Network (SIGN) published SIGN 55, which gives guidance on the care of adults and children with diabetes. This was followed in 2002 by the Scottish Diabetes Framework (Scottish Executive Health Department, 2002).

This document set out 7 'first stage priority issues':
- Information, education, and empowerment.
- Heart disease.
- Eye care.
- Strategy, leadership, and team working.
- Education and training for professionals.
- IM&T and diabetes registers.
- Implementation and monitoring.

The Scottish Diabetes Group, a multi-disciplinary advisory group was set up to monitor and support the implementation of the Scottish Diabetes Framework.

An annual report, the Scottish Diabetes Survey, is also published by this group.

In 2003, there are plans to extend the digital retinopathy screening programme to cover all people over 12 years of age in Scotland.

The Scottish Executive published *Delivering Health* in 2005, a programme for NHS action in Scotland. This document highlights the value of improving the management of the care for people with long-term conditions and gives diabetes care as an example.

More information may be obtained from 🖥 www.scotpho.org.uk/home/Healthwell-beinganddisease/Diabetes/diabetes_policy.asp

Throughout the UK

In 2004 contractual changes for all UK GPs provided a set of quality indicators within a Quality and Outcomes Framework (QOF). These indicators were revised in 2006 to include 18 indicators for diabetes care generating information regarding diabetes and offering significant incentives to improve care delivery.

This is downloadable in a PDF format from 🖥 www.dh.gov.uk/en/Healthcare/Primarycare/Primarycarecontracting/QOF/DH_4125653

Diabetes policy: Wales

The Welsh Assembly published NSF Standards for Diabetes Care in 2002 followed with a Delivery Strategy in 2003. Copies of these can be obtained from 🖥 www.wales.gov.uk.

Diabetes policy: Northern Ireland

The Joint Task Force on diabetes was established in 2001 and was charged with producing a framework for the delivery of care in Northern Ireland. Their report, *A Blueprint for Diabetes Care in Northern Ireland*, was presented to Clinical Resources Efficiency Support Team (CREST) and Diabetes UK in 2003. Covering 5 key areas, comprising 18 building blocks:

Prevention and early detection
- Health promotion.
- Public education.
- Screening high risk groups.
- Community issues, groups, and interagency working.

Care monitoring and treatment
- Education for people with diabetes and health professionals.
- Eye screening.
- Integrated diabetes care and guidelines.
- Emotional and psychological support.

Targeting vulnerable groups
- Children and young people.
- Ethnic minority communities.
- Pregnancy and sexual health.
- Other vulnerable groups.

Planning and managing services
- Strategy, leadership, and team working.
- Workforce planning.
- Information management and diabetes registers.
- User forum and empowerment.
- Audit, research, and development.

Implementation
- Implementation and monitoring.

Diabetes policy: Republic of Ireland

In 2002, the Diabetes Service Development Group report, *Diabetes care: securing the future*, was published in the Republic of Ireland. The report can be viewed at 🖳 http://www. diabetes.ie/website/content/diabetes_in_ireland/dsdg-report.aspx.

Chapter 17

Health education

Resources

The NSF for diabetes states:

> Structured education can improve knowledge, blood glucose control, weight and dietary management, physical activity and psychological well-being, particularly when this is tailored to the needs of the individual and includes skills-based approaches to education (p. 2)

Health education can be seen as one of the basic tools that underpin patient empowerment and NICE recommend that a structured programme of education is provided for patients from the time of their diagnosis onwards. In order to provide this the Department of Health (DoH) has recognized the necessity of having a professional work force that is well informed and educated in the latest developments of care for people with diabetes.

Modules containing diabetes educational material are available for professional development and may be downloaded from 🖳 www.idf.org/home/index.cfm?=503

There are many resources available for patient education and it is important to consider their origin and accuracy. Those provided by the DoH or National Institute for Health and Clinical Excellence (NICE) are utilized as examples within this section.

Principles

NICE recognizes the paucity of evidence available with which to assess different models of education and their effectiveness. However, they have produced guidance on good principles of education:

- Educational interventions should reflect established principles of adult learning (e.g. be experiential).
- Education should be provided by an appropriately trained multidisciplinary team.
- Decisions regarding the appropriateness of group work versus individual teaching and group sessions should be accessible to the broadest range of people.
- Educational programmes should use a variety of techniques to promote learning styles for people with diabetes.
- Education should be an integrated part of long-term, routine, diabetes care.

The full document, *Technological appraisal 60* (issue date 2003), may be accessed from 🖳 www.nice.org.uk or by telephoning 0870 1555 455 quoting ref. no. 213

The National Diabetes Support Team, provide a leaflet for patients to enable them to assess the delivery of education that they are offered. They suggest a good planned education course should:
- Provide a written outline.
- Be delivered by trained educators.
- Be quality assured.

DAFNE for those with Type 1 diabetes and DESMOND for those with Type 2 are given as examples of programmes that meet the key criteria for structured education.

Further information

Dose Adjustment for Normal Eating (DAFNE) 🖳 www.dafne.uk.com

Diabetes Education and Self Management for Ongoing and Newly Diagnosed 🖳 www.desmond-project.org.uk

Diabetes UK has produced structured education support tools. Available as a downloadable PDF from: 🖳 www.diabetes.org.uk/Documents/Professionals/toolkits/Toolkit%20handbook.doc

DoH has published *Living with diabetes: your future health and wellbeing.* If you require copies of this publication quote 29335 *Living with Diabetes: your future health and wellbeing* and contact:: Department of Health Publications, PO Box 777, London SE1 6XH, UK. Tel: 08701 555 455. Fax: 01623 724524. E-mail doh@prolog.uk.com. 08700 102870 – Textphone (for minicom users) for the hard of hearing (open 08.00–18.00 Monday to Friday). This publication is also available on request in Braille, on audio cassette, CD, in large print, and in other languages. It is also available on the department's website at: 🖳 www.dh.gov.uk/en/Healthcare/NationalServiceFrameworks/Diabetes/index.htm

Screening

This section is considered in 2 parts:
- Screening the population for Type 2 diabetes.
- Screening people with diabetes for complications.

Screening the population for Type 2 diabetes

David Lammy, the Health Minister in 2003, stressed the importance that 'people at risk of developing the disease (Type 2 diabetes) are identified before they develop the symptoms'.

In 2003, 9 inner city pilot sites were set up, where GP's used BG measurement to screen people at risk of developing diabetes.

Those screened included
- Those over 40 years of age.
- The overweight.
- Those who have heart disease.
- Those who have had a stroke.

An example of this proactive screening is the Department of Health pilot project undertaken by Slough PCT, which aimed at finding people from ethnic minority backgrounds who are undiagnosed, but have diabetes. As many as 7% of the population in Slough already have diabetes and this project is about reducing late diagnosis of the disease and improving the health of those most at risk.

Practice-based disease registers are at the heart of proactive screening as they may be used to identify those potentially at risk.

NB. The National Screening Committee Policy Position in July 2006 recommended that general population screening for diabetes should not be undertaken as it failed to meet several of their criteria.

Screening people with diabetes for complications

The NSF helps people know what to expect from diabetes services. As a minimum, every year, people should expect:
- To be checked for early signs of complications that can be treated:
  - diabetic retinopathy;
  - diabetic nephropathy;
  - diabetic neuropathy;
  - cardiovascular disease, including coronary heart disease, stroke and transient ischemic attacks, and peripheral vascular disease.

Guidance on vascular risk assessment screening is currently being considered by the UK National Screening Committee (NSC).

Other conditions occur more commonly in people with diabetes and should be noted on assessment:
- Cataracts (occur 10 years earlier and are twice as common in people with diabetes).
- Urinary tract and skin infections.
- Frozen shoulder and trigger finger.
- Mental health problems, such as depression or eating disorders.
- Skin diseases specific to diabetes (see 📖 Skin conditions, p. 216).

Raising public awareness

Diabetes UK estimate that 19% of people with diabetes are undiagnosed or not recorded on general practice registers.

Local, regional, national, and international campaigns have been instigated to raise the awareness of the population as a whole to aspects of living with, risk factors for, and signs and symptoms of diabetes (Table 17.1). This is done to prevent delay in diagnosis and treatment for people with Type 2 diabetes and thus reduce their risks of developing complications associated with high concentrations of BG.

Various resources have been used to bring diabetes to the forefront of the collective consciousness. The United Nations (UN, 2006) promoted an annual World Diabetes Day, on the 14th November, to raise global awareness.

Diabetes UK ran a 'measure up campaign', which focused public attention on the implications of having a waist circumference greater than 37"(94cm) for men and 31.5"(80cm) for women. A combination of posters, online targeting of at risk groups, local newspaper advertisements, and a road show offering a simple 2min test, was offered in 20 localities over a period of 1year. In addition, lobbying of elected representatives was undertaken by raising their awareness though a poster campaign aimed at the Houses of Parliament and campaigning at political party conferences.

Radio Ramadan-Bradford City tPCt linked up with GPs, health professionals, and patients, and broadcast a series of health education programmes designed for the Asian community over the 4 week period of Ramadan (16 October–15 November). All programmes on Iqra 87.7FM are in Urdu/English and on Radio Sabrang in Punjabi.

Further information

United Nations General Assembly (2006) Resolution Adopted by the General Assembly – 61/225, World Diabetes Day. UN General Assembly, New York.

Table 17.1 Risk factors for developing Type 2 diabetes

Risk factor	Specifically
Obesity	Raised BMI – (calculator online ▣ http://www.diabetes.co.uk/bmi.html)
Sedentary life style	Increasing exercise helps: • Control weight • Make insulin utilization more effective • Decreases insulin resistance
Abdominal obesity (waist measurements)	For all women, a waist measurement of over 80cm (31.5in) indicates increased risk For all white or black men, a waist measurement of over 94cm (37in) indicates increased risk For Asian men, a waist measurement of over 90cm (35in) indicates increased risk
Age	Over 40 Over 25 if you're black or Asian
Metabolic syndrome	Metabolic syndrome is present if there is evidence of any 3 of the following: • Increased waist circumference ($\geq$102cm in men and $\geq$88cm in women; $\geq$90cm in Asian men and $\geq$80cm in Asian women), indicating central obesity • Elevated triglycerides ($\geq$1.7mmol/l) • Decreased HDL cholesterol <1.03mmol/l for men, <1.29mmol/l for women) • Blood pressure >130/85mmHg or having active treatment for hypertension • Fasting plasma glucose level >5.6mmol/l or active treatment for hyperglycaemia
Genetic	Have a close family member (parent, brother or sister) with Type 2 diabetes South Asian or African-Caribbean (these ethnic groups are five times more likely to get Type 2 diabetes)
Other associated conditions-	Polycystic ovary syndrome (PCOS), especially if also overweight following gestational diabetes Ischaemic heart disease, cerebrovascular disease, peripheral vascular disease, hypertension

Clinical governance

Models of clinical governance

Background

Scally and Donaldson (1998) describe clinical governance (CG) as:

> ...the main vehicle for continuously improving the quality of patient care and developing the capacity of the NHS in England to maintain high standards (including dealing with poor professional performance). (p. 61)

The Royal College of Nursing (RCN, 1998) describes CG as:

> ...a framework through which NHS organizations are accountable for continuously improving the quality of their services and safeguarding high standards of care by creating an environment in which excellence in clinical care will flourish.

The following NHS reforms launched CG in the 1990s in each of the 4 home countries:

- Department of Health (1997) *The new NHS: modern, dependable.* HMSO, London.
- Department of Health, Social Services and Public Safety (2001) *Best practice – best care.* DHSSPS, Belfast.
- Scottish Executive (1997) *Designed to care: renewing the National Health Service in Scotland.* Scottish Executive Health Department, Edinburgh.
- Welsh Office (1998) *NHS Wales; putting patients first.* National Assembly for Wales, Cardiff.

Models

Principles of CG originate from corporate governance, developed to address poor standards in the business world and later expanded to embrace public services, including the NHS and private sector health care delivery. Clinical governance requires creativity and leadership across each healthcare institution to facilitate improvements in standards through locally developed programmes (see ☐ Evidence bases for best practice, p. 340), which cover the following areas:

- Universalize practice.
- Consolidate practice.
- Codify practice.
- Demonstrate accountability.

Tools to facilitate CG in practice include:

- Clinical audit.
- Risk management.
- Evidence-based practice and clinical effectiveness guidance.
- Learning from adverse events/complaints/incidents.
- Providing evidence of:
  - continuous professional development (CPD) and leadership;
  - strategic planning and service review.

The World Health Organization's (WHO) model divides CG into 4 areas

- Professional performance – technical quality.
- Resource use – efficiency.
- Risk management – risk of injury/illness associated with service provided.
- Patients' satisfaction with the service provided.

The RCN suggests CG areas are

- Patient focus – how services are based on patient needs.
- Information focus – how information is used.
- Quality improvement – how standards are reviewed and attained.
- Staff focus – how staff are developed.
- Leadership – how improvement efforts are planned.
- Clinical audit.
- Staff development.
- Clinical effectiveness.
- Clinical risk management.
- Clinical audit.
- Evidence-based practice.

Further information

Cadbury Committee (1992) *Report of the Committee on the Financial Aspects of Corporate Governance.* Gee and Co., London.

Royal College of Nursing (1998) *Clinical Governance: an RCN resource guide.* Available at ▣ www. rcn.org.uk (accessed 1st June 2009).

Scally, G., Donaldson, L.J. (1998) Clinical governance and the drive for quality improvement in the new NHS in England. *Br Med J* **317**, 61–5.

Scottish Executive (1997) *Designed to care: renewing the National Health Service in Scotland.* Scottish Executive Health Department, Edinburgh.

World Health Organization (1983) *The principles of quality assurance.* WHO, Copenhagen. Available at: ▣ www.rcn.org.uk (accessed 20th December 2008).

Courses

Clinical governance was introduced in 1997 as a result of the Department of Health's White Paper *A First Class Service*, which placed a new duty of demonstrating quality on all health organizations in the UK. Potentially, it can ensure high standards of clinical care are maintained throughout the country. Each of the three models outlined include staff development/ trading as an important area of CG and specifically leadership.

Examples of course providers:

- The RCN offers a range of leadership and team development programmes for members and health care organizations. These include bespoke programmes developed with organizations to meet specific organizational needs and the RCN Clinical Leadership Programme. Contact the team on Tel: 020 7647 3836.
- The National Prescribing Centre (NPC) also offer training packages at ⊡ www.npc.co.uk
- The Clinical Governance Support team offer training and workshops around the following aspects of CG:
  - patient experience
  - board development
  - primary care
  - international healthcare development
  - team coach and patient safety
  - publications
  - web sites
  - IT support.

Details can be found at ⊡ www.appraisalsupport.nhs.uk

Two external bodies facilitate and reinforce the local responsibility for quality programmes:

- Commissioner for Health Improvement (CHI).
- National Institute for Health and Clinical Excellence (NIHCE).

Continuous professional development

Health care practice and delivery are constantly changing and nurses have a statutory obligation to maintain and develop their competency through a lifelong learning process called continuous professional development (CPD).

The link between CPD and the delivery of quality care has been explicitly made in the following professional body, government, and regulatory body documents:

- Scottish Executive Health Department (1999) *Learning together: a strategy for education, training, lifelong learning for the NHS in Scotland.* SEHD, Edinburgh.
- DoH (1999) *A first class service.* HMSO, London.
- DoH (2000) *Improving working lives standard.* HMSO, London.
- DoH (2000) *The NHS Plan: a plan for investment a plan for reform.* HMSO, London.
- DoH (2004) *NHS knowledge and skills framework (NHS KSF) and the development and review process.* HMSO, London.
- Welsh Assembly Government (WAG)(2006) *Designed for life: quality requirements in adult critical care.* Health and Social Care Department, Cardiff.
- Health Professions Council (HPC) (2005) *Standards for continuing development.* HPC, London.

CPD needs are identified through:
- Daily reflection on practice.
- Clinical supervision and appraisal.
- Personal development plans (PDPs)

Statutory requirements in addition to CPD include:
- The Health and Safety at Work Act 1974.
- The Data Protection Legislation Act.

The Nursing and Midwifery Council (NMC) Code of Professional Conduct (2008) states that, as a registered nurse, you must:
- Keep your skills and knowledge up to date.
- You must have the knowledge and skills for safe and effective practice when working without direct supervision.
- You must recognize and work within the limits of your competence.
- You must take part in appropriate learning and practice activities that maintain and develop your competence and performance.

Sources of help and support with CPD

Nationally
- National Electronic Library for Health (NELH).
- Professional organizations.
- National Library of Guidelines Specialist Library ⌨ www.library.nhs.uk/ GuidelinesFinder

Locally
- Health care libraries in local universities and on health care premises.
- In-house and Trust training.

Evidence bases for best practice

Evidence-based practice refers to assessing and appraising evidence for use when making clinical or care delivery decisions. Clinical appraisal is the skill of assessing and interpreting evidence by systematically considering:
- Results.
- Validity.
- Relevance.
- Source.

Classification of evidence

Evidence within the NSF's are classified according to source with studies from research methods listed in 1, yielding the strongest evidence and 4 the weakest:
1 Meta-analyses, systematic reviews of randomized controlled trials (RCTs), including cluster RCTs.
2 Systematic reviews of or individual non-randomized controlled trials, case-control studies, cohort studies, controlled before and after studies (CBA), interrupted time series studies (ITS), correlation studies.
3 Non-analytical studies, e.g. case reports.
4 Expert opinion.

Clinical appraisal of clinical evidence is becoming a core competency and CG will require professionals to recognize and use elements of good practice in other areas to enhance care delivery in their own area.

Useful sources

It is important to consider the origin of any information under consideration. The following sites provide reviewed evidence.
- NICE (🖳 www.NICE.org.uk).
- NHS electronic library for health (NLH), diabetes specialist library (🖳 www.library.nhs.uk/diabetes/Page.aspx?pagename=AEU07).
- Cochrane (🖳 www.cochrane.org).
- National Service Framework (NSF) for Diabetes (🖳 www.dh.gov.uk).
- National Diabetes Support Team (🖳 www.diabetes.nhs.uk).
- Diabetes UK (🖳 www.diabetes.org.uk).
- Public Health Observatory in Diabetes (🖳 www.yhpho.org.uk)
- *British Medical Journal* summary of updated NICE guideline on the management of type 2 diabetes (🖳 http://www.bmj.com/cgi/content/extract/336/7656/1306).
- Database of uncertainties about the effects of treatments (DUETs): a resource to help prioritize new research (🖳 www.library.nhs.uk/DUETs).

Case studies

Introduction to the case studies

This section contains six fictitious vignettes containing approaches to care for patients with specific needs. Whilst it is always important to follow the protocols or guidelines used in the area in which you work, the following are an attempt to put theory into practical examples. The answers given following the vignettes, although following good practice guidelines, not definitive answers. It is important to always be aware of and follow locally agreed guidelines and health care plans.

Vignette 1: person newly diagnosed with Type 2 diabetes

Mrs Martin is 51 years old and has been newly diagnosed with Type 2 diabetes. Her visit to the surgery was prompted by her anxiety regarding increasing polydypsia and lethargy. Her fasting BG level was 7.8mmol/l; this alongside her symptoms is diagnostic of Type 2 diabetes.

Mrs Martin's HbA1c on diagnosis is 7.9% and her weight is 90kg with a BMI of 31.

She has few concerns about her weight, but in discussion regarding her present eating patterns, she described a diet that was based on refined carbohydrates. Apart from a 5min stroll from the car park to her work place and housework she did no additional exercise. Her father, a person with Type 2 diabetes, had required a below knee amputation of his right leg many years before, and so Mrs Martin is both anxious and well motivated to make any lifestyle changes needed to reduce her risk of complications.

How might you proceed?

Vignette 2: person with Type 2 diabetes

Mr Parsons, a 40 year-old ex-rugby player, has very recently been diagnosed with Type 2 diabetes. He weighs 140.3kg, has a BMI of 36.3, his bp is 167/98mmol/l Hg, and his HbA1c is 9%. He is a smoker with a sedentary occupation and takes little exercise each week.

He described his social life, which includes heavy drinking at the village rugby club with his old team mates every weekend and, on average, one additional evening a week. He estimates his alcohol intake at well over double the DoH recommendations.

Department of health recommendations for alcohol intake for a man

The regular consumption of between 3 and 4 units a day for men of all ages will not accrue significant health risk.

Four units equates to under 2pints of 4% beer (4.4 units) and just over 1.5pints of 5% beer (4.2 units).

Although Mr Parsons had no specific symptoms caused by his diabetes, a discussion of the risk factors engendered by his present life style is required.

How might you proceed?

Vignette 3: person with increased risk of developing diabetes

Mrs Nisha Patel had been prompted to visit a diabetes testing stall, run by the local diabetes specialist team at a local community event, as she had been gradually putting on weight around her middle. There she had her finger pricked and a random BG estimation made. Her random BG was elevated, but not in the diabetic range. Mrs Patel is 48 years of age and she was advised to visit her surgery for a fasting BG test, and some more advice regarding weight loss and the chance to join an Asian slimming project. Why might this have been?

Vignette 4: person newly diagnosed with Type 1 diabetes

John Richardson is a usually fit and active 17 year-old, and a student at a sixth form college. John plays cricket and cycles to college, some 6 miles from his home each day. He has visited his general practice as he was feeling extremely tired, thirsty, and was passing a lot of urine. He had presumed this was because he was drinking a lot of lemonade to quench his thirst. He is living at home with his mother, father, and two younger brothers. He has lost a considerable amount of weight over the past month without reducing his food intake or increasing his exercise. His random laboratory BG is 16.5mmol/l, and his urine has a trace of ketones

How should John's care proceed?

Vignette 5: person with increased risk of gestational diabetes

Mandy, a 28 year-old mother of two, is delighted to discover she is weeks into her third pregnancy. Her two sons, Tyler and Marshall, aged 5 and 3 respectively, are thriving. Mandy was diagnosed with gestational diabetes during her pregnancy with Marshall. Her BMI is 31 and she smokes at least 10 cigarettes a day, but would describe herself as being in good health and active with the care of her sons and home. She does not work outside the home. Her grandmother was diagnosed with Type 2 diabetes when she was 56 years of age. How might you proceed with Mandy's pre-natal care?

Vignette 6: person at increased risk of Type 2 diabetes

Mrs Andrews was struggling to lose her post-pregnancy weight gain. Her BMI was now 43 and she reported that her ideal weight would be 63.5kg and was overwhelmed and tearful when told her present weight was 107.95kg. Having had gestational diabetes in her pregnancy she is at high risk of developing Type 2 diabetes in the future.

She had tried 'every diet in the book' without success.

Her usual eating patterns included takeaway fast food on most days of the week as she often felt too exhausted to cook for herself and partner after cooking several different meals for the children. Mr and Mrs Andrews usually ate late at night and Mrs Andrews would often eat leftover food from the children's plates earlier in the evening.

How might you proceed?

Possible answer: vignette 1

Mrs Martin, age 51 years, with newly-diagnosed Type 2 diabetes

Following discussion, some dietary changes were agreed upon to reduce the refined carbohydrate content of her diet and by doing this to improve her BG levels. The National Institute for Health and Clinical Excellence (NICE) published May 2008 recommends a diet based on energy intake with 55–60% carbohydrate, 15–20% protein, and 20–30% fat as evidence shows such a diet can produce a modest improvement in glycaemic control. This involved:

- Starting to use artificial sweetener in hot drinks in place of sugar.
- Having wholegrain cereal for breakfast.
- Swapping carbonated drinks to the sugar-free varieties.
- NICE (2008) recommends metformin at diagnosis.

It may be the practice in your area to refer Mrs Martin immediately to a dietician for advice. As with all the advice given in this handbook it is important to follow local guidelines.

Contact details and informative literature was given to support the information discussed. In the area where Mrs Martin lives, it is the practice to teach her how to monitor and record her BG levels. She can be loaned a BG meter, and issued with a finger pricker and lancets. A prescription for blood testing strips was issued and a follow-up appointment made for 8weeks.

For reference see 📖 Structured education: meeting NICE criteria, p. 106; 📖 Exercise, p. 268.

Possible answer: vignette 2

Mr Parsons, age 40 years, with established Type 2 diabetes

It is imperative that any plan of action is mutually agreed. First, it was decided to tackle his smoking as he already wanted to quit, both because of the expense and family pressures. Mr Parsons had a PC at home and so the NHS Smokefree website was recommended as a resource as it has lots of advice and contacts offering a four-step approach of:

- Get ready.
- Make a plan.
- Go smoke free.
- Keep going.

He was also enrolled in the local surgery quit smoking group, where he discussed the use of nicotine patches, gum, or the use of buproprion with his practice nurse.

Mr Parsons was taught how to monitor his BG levels and issued with the equipment required to this. Guidelines from NICE/EASD/ADA suggest that he should be started on metformin immediately.

The second step of his plan involved addressing his alcohol intake with a view to reducing it to safer levels. Mr Parsons also made the suggestion that, by reducing the number and length of times he went out for a drink, he would reduce the number of times when his temptation to smoke was at its highest.

Contact numbers and times were given in case he had further questions or needed advice, and a follow-up visit was planned for 1month later to see how he was progressing and to review his BG monitoring.

One month on

Mr Parsons had managed to stop smoking with the help of the support group. He had also reduced his alcohol intake by half without feeling deprived. Because of this change, his weight had reduced by 3kg. Although he ate a healthy diet, it was decided that he and his wife would visit the dietitian to discuss any changes that could be made to his portion sizes and meal plans. His home BG monitoring showed a slight decrease in levels with pre-prandial readings of 8–9mmol/l and post-prandial glucose of 10–11mmol/l. His morning fasting glucose was 8mmol/l. Mr Parsons decided to continue monitoring his BG levels for another month, whilst carrying out any recommendations made by the dietitian. Although the UKPDS 38 (1998) showed that 23% of patients initially achieved fasting BG levels below 7.8mmol/l without pharmacological intervention, the 2008 NICE guidelines recommend commencing metformin at the first visit.

Further information

UK Prospective Diabetes Study (UKPDS) Group (1998). Tight blood pressure control and risk of macrovascular and microvasular complications in type 2 diabetes: UKPDS 38. *BMJ* **317**, 703–13.

Possible answer: vignette 3

Mrs Patel, age 48 years, in a pre-diabetic state

NICE guidelines for Type 2 diabetes (🖥 www.nice.org.uk) refer to metabolic syndrome, which they list as a combination of:

- Insulin insensitivity.
- Excess body weight or obesity, especially abdominal adiposity (increased waist circumference).
- The weight gain is exacerbated by over-eating and lack of exercise.
- Raised bp.
- Abnormal blood fat profile.
- Increased risk of diabetes in the Asian community.

Diabetes UK are, at present, running a campaign to raise awareness of the risk to metabolism of carrying too much weight around the waistline. They quote research as showing that a large waist could mean an individual is up to 12 times more likely to develop diabetes.

They suggest the at-risk waist measurements are 37in (94cm) or more for men, except those of South Asian origin who are at risk at 35in (88.9cm) or more, and 31.5in (80cm) or more for all women.

The National Diabetes Information Clearing House (NDIC) available at 🖥 http://diabetes.niddk.nih.gov/dm/pubs/insulinresistance/index.htm offers simple advice regarding what may be called 'the pre-diabetic state'. This site explains the link between insulin resistance, the pre-diabetic state, and Type 2 diabetes.

Mrs Patel underwent a fasting glucose: this result was 6.1mmol/l, which indicated impaired fasting glycaemia (IFT). She was offered lifestyle advice, which covered dietary recommendations for weight loss, exercise advice, and referral to her local Asian weight loss clinic. Diabetes UK recommends rescreening Mrs Patel annually or earlier if a clinical need arises. They have produced a useful leaflet for health professionals as part of their 'Measure up' campaign. It is available from: 🖥 www.diabetes.org.uk

Note: other definitions of similar conditions have been developed by the World Health Organization and the Association of Clinical Endocrinologists.

Further information

National Cholesterol Education Program, Third Report of the Expert Panel on Detection, Evaluation, and Treatment of High Blood Cholesterol in Adults (Adult Treatment Panel III), National Heart, Lung, and Blood Institute, National Institutes of Health, May 2001.

Possible answer: vignette 4

John Richardson, age 17 years, newly diagnosed with Type 1 diabetes

NICE guidelines (2004) recommend the use of the World Health Organization 1999 report on the diagnosis and classification of diabetes mellitus. This lists the signs and symptoms of Type 1 diabetes as:

- Polyuria.
- Polydypsia.
- Weight loss.
- Blood glucose more than 11mmol/l.
- Ketonuria.

John is displaying the classic symptoms of Type 1 diabetes and NICE recommend **immediate referral** to a multidisciplinary care team. The team will provide him with training in the following areas (see 📖 Chapter 6, pp. 105–118):

- Clinical care of his condition.
- Education regarding life style choices.
- Foot care advice and assessment.
- Nutrition advice and assessment.

Home-based management of care will be ideal for John as he is not ketotic. John will need to be shown how to:

- Undertake a capillary BG estimation using a meter.
- How to give an injection of insulin. Given his lifestyle a basal bolus insulin regime may be the most appropriate.

John's ongoing education will include topics such as:

- The aims of insulin therapy.
- Delivery methods for insulin.
- Self-monitoring of BG.
- How to react to fluctuations in BG levels.
- The effect of diet/physical activity.
- How to deal with intercurrent illness.
- Detection and management of hypoglycaemia.

Possible answer: vignette 5

Mandy, age 28 years, with a previous history of gestational diabetes

NICE guidelines identify the following risk factors for developing gestational diabetes:

- Body mass index above 30kg/m^2.
- Previous macrosomic baby (weighing 4.5kg or above).
- Previous gestational diabetes.
- Family history of diabetes (first-degree relative with diabetes).
- Family origin with a high prevalence of diabetes.
- South Asian (specifically women whose country of family origin is India, Pakistan, or Bangladesh).
- Black Caribbean.
- Middle Eastern, specifically women whose country of family origin is:
  - Saudi Arabia, United Arab Emirates;
  - Iraq, Jordan, Syria, Oman, Qatar;
  - Kuwait, Lebanon, Egypt.

(NICE, 2008, p. 15).

Mandy has three of the risk factors for developing gestational diabetes and NICE recommends that screening be carried out using a 2h 75g oral glucose tolerance test (OGTT) and the diagnostic criteria recommended by the World Health Organization (WHO). A 2h plasma venous glucose equal to or greater then 7.8mmol/l.

NICE suggest this test be offered at 16–18 weeks gestation to women who have and gestational diabetes at an earlier pregnancy. If the first test results are within normal parameters a second test should be offered at 28weeks.

NICE do not recommend screening for these women using a fasting plasma glucose, a random BG, a glucose challenge test, or urinalysis for glucose.

Mandy should be reminded of the importance of maintaining good glycaemic control during her pregnancy for the sake of her own and her baby's health.

NICE notes that untreated hyperglycaemia during pregnancy may result in a macrocosmic baby, trauma to the mother and/or baby during delivery, neonatal hypoglycaemia or perinatal death. It may also predispose to delivery by caesarean section (NICE 2008a, p. 17).

Mandy should be shown how to monitor her BG and issued with the appropriate equipment. The BG targets are the same for Mandy as for women with diabetes at the time of becoming pregnant. If it is safe to do so, bearing in mind risks from hypoglycaemia, pre-prandial BG should be in the range of 3.5–5.9mmol/l and a 1h post-prandial BG level below 7.8mmol/l should be maintained throughout pregnancy.

NB: HbA1c estimations should not be used to assess glycaemic control during the second and third trimesters of pregnancy.

To ensure tight glycaemic control and smooth glucose release dietary considerations should include:

- Carbohydrates with a low GI should be chosen.
- Carbohydrate intake should be restricted to 25kcal/km/day or less as Mandy's BMI is over 25kg/m² (NICE, 2008a).
- Lean meat.
- Oily fish.
- A balance between polyunsaturated and monounsaturated fats.
- Moderate exercise for at least 30min each day should be undertaken.

If it does not prove possible to control Mandy's BG parameters within the target range hypoglycaemic medication will be require, which is tailored to the glucose profile and is acceptable to Mandy.

During her last pregnancy Mandy used a rapid-acting insulin analogue during the last trimester of her pregnancy, and if her BG levels do not respond to dietary restrictions and exercise this may be considered for her again.

Mandy's care during her routine antenatal care should be given bearing in mind the NICE Clinical Guideline 62, 2008b).

She should be given advice and support regarding stopping smoking (see 📖 p. 288), which is extremely risky, both for the complications of diabetes and her pregnancy.

Further information

National Institute of Clinical Excellence (2008a) *Diabetes in pregnancy. management of diabetes and its complications from pre-conception to post natal period*, NICE Clinical Guideline 63. NICE, London. Available at: 🖥 www.nice.org.uk/nicemedia/pdf/CG063NICEGuideline.pdf (accessed 18th March 2009)

National Institute of Clinical Excellence (2008b) *NICE Clinical Guideline 62*. NICE, London. Available at: 🖥 www.nice.org.uk/CG062 (accessed 18th March 2009).

Possible answer: vignette 6

Mrs Andrews, in a pre-diabetic state

Following discussion, Mrs Andrews agreed to commence pharmaco-therapy (refer to local guidelines or protocols) and reduced her consumption of fast food to twice a week. An appointment was made to support and further discuss any progress for 2 weeks later.

On visiting the surgery 2 weeks later, the changes Mrs Andrews had carried out were discussed in light of the behaviour change information provided by the pharmaceutical company.

A second appointment was made for 1 month later and Mrs Andrews had lost 10lb in weight and dropped a dress size. She was delighted with her success and other small changes in her previous eating patterns were negotiated to continue the weight loss.

Three months later, Mrs Andrews had lost 2 stone and her BMI was now 38. This was achieved by reducing her takeaway meals to 1 a month, eating earlier in the evening, and walking to and from school with the children each day. This easily enabled her to achieve 30min of exercise 5 times a week.

The Diabetes Prevention Programme research study of 3234 people showed that moderate dietary changes, regular exercise and a 5–7% weight loss can delay and prevent Type 2 diabetes. The results showed that people in the lifestyle change group with an average weight loss of 15lbs in the first year, reduced their risk of getting Type 2 diabetes by 58%. Lifestyle change was even more effective in those aged 60 and older who reduced their risk by 71%.

More information regarding the Diabetes Prevention Programme can be found on the National Diabetes Information Clearing House website (🖥 http://diabetes.niddk.nih.gov/dm/pubs/preventionprogram/).

A further review of studies (Wild and Byrne, 2006) has reported that every kilogram of weight loss is associated with the following changes in lipid concentrations:
• Fasting serum cholesterol: 1.0%.
• Low density lipoprotein (LDL) cholesterol: 0.7%.
• Triglycerides: 1.9%.
• HDL cholesterol: 0.2%.

Further information

Wild SH, Byrne CD. (2006) Risk factors for diabetes and coronary heart disease. *Br Med J*; **333**, 1009–11.

Glossary

Acetone The simplest ketone.

Acidosis A metabolic condition, characterized by an increase in hydrogen ion concentration, that occurs when the body is no longer able to buffer free hydrogen ions in the blood, resulting from either the accumulation of acid or depletion of the alkaline reserve (bicarbonate) in the blood and body tissues. This usually causes the pH of the blood to drop (and become more acidic).

Acromegaly A condition that results from the excess production of growth hormone in the anterior lobe of the pituitary gland. Acromegaly is characterized by enlarged facial features, enlarged jaw, enlarged frontal bone of skull, widely spaced teeth, and enlargement of the bones of the extremities.

Acuity Clarity of vision or hearing.

Adipose tissue Connective tissue modified to store fat.

Adrenergic The release of adrenaline.

Albuminuria Protein in the urine.

Alpha cells Specialized cells in pancreas that secrete glucagon.

Angioplasty Repair of a blood vessel.

Atherosclerosis Progressive hardening and narrowing of the arteries over a life.

Auto-immune A disease process that involves the production of host antibodies to host tissue.

Base A chemical term for a substance that combines with an acid to form a salt.

C-peptide C-peptide is a by-product of normal insulin production by the beta cells in the pancreas.

Carbohydrate Collective term for all forms of starch and sugar.

Cataract Opacity of the lens of the eye impao.

Catecholamine Catecholamines include adrenaline, noradrenaline, and dopamine, with roles as hormones and neurotransmitters.

Chromosome Self-replicating genetic structure of a cell containg the DNA.

Coeliac disease Sensitivity to gluten causes the villi in the gut to atrophy, impairing the absorption of nutrients.

Connective tissue Specialized mesodermally derived tissue.

Counter regulatory A substance giving an equal and opposite reaction, e.g insulin and glucagon.

Cushings An increased concentration of glucocorticoid hormone (ACTH) in the bloodstream, Symptoms include weight gain, central obesity, moon face, weakness, fatigue, backache, headache, increased thirst, increased urination, impotence, mental status changes, and muscle atrophy.

Endocrine Internal hormone secretions.

Endogenous Developing or originating within the organ.

Epinephrine A synonym for adrenaline. A hormone produced by the adrenal medulla in mammals. It can be produced synthetically for medical purposes. It is secreted by the adrenal medulla in response to low blood glucose, exercise and stress, and causes a breakdown of glycogen to glucose in the liver, encourages the release of fatty acids from adipose tissue, causes vasodilation of the small arteries within muscle, and increases cardiac output.

Exocrine External secretions via a duct.

Fundoscopy Examination of the retina, optic disc, and blood vessels of the eye.

Gastroparesis A condition where there is delayed stomach emptying (due to abnormal gastric motility).

Gene Unit of heredity to be found on a chromosome.

Genotype The genetic make up of an organism or a cell.

Glucagon A hormone produced by the alpha cells in the pancreas, responsible for raising blood glucose levels.

Gluconeogenisis The formation of new glucose from stored glucose.

Gluten Wheat protein.

Glycogen The form in which carbohydrate is stored.

Glycogenolysis The breakdown of glycogen to glucose.

HbA1c Measurement of blood glucose control, measures glucose attachment to glycated haemoglobin over the previous 8–12 weeks.

HDL These lipoproteins acts to carry cholesterol in the bloodstream.

Hepatic Pertaining to the liver.

Hyperglycaemia High blood glucose level.

Hyperinsulinaemia High blood insulin level.

Hyperlipdaemia High blood levels of fat.

Hyperosmolar An increase in the osmotic concentration of a solution. A complication seen in diabetes mellitus in which very marked hyperglycaemia occur causing osmotic shifts in water in brain cells and resulting in coma. It can be fatal or lead to permanent neurological damage. Ketoacidosis does not occur in these cases.

Hypoglycaemia Low blood glucose levels.

Hypothalamic Of or involving the hypothalamus.

Hypothalamus A portion of the brain that lies beneath the thalamus and secretes substances, which control metabolism by exerting an influence on pituitary gland function. The hypothalamus is involved in the regulation of body temperature, water balance, blood sugar, and fat metabolism. It also regulates other glands, such as the ovaries, parathyroids, and thyroid.

Insulitis Inflammation of the islets of Langerhans, with lymphocytic infiltration, which may result from viral infection and be the initial lesion of insulin-dependent diabetes mellitus.

Intermittent claudication Pain in the calves relieved by rest.

Islet cell antibodies Antibodies to the islet cells. The presence of ICA combined with a decrease in the first-phase of insulin secretion is predictive with a 95% likelihood of the development of insulin-dependent diabetes mellitus within 12 months.

Islets of Langerhans Cells within the pancreas that secrete insulin and glucagon.

Ketoacidosis A serious condition related to a lack of insulin, which causes the use of fat for energy, this results in ketone formation and acidosis, signs include ketones in urine, hyperglycaemia, vomiting, and altered state of consciousness.

Ketogenisis The formation of ketones.

Ketones By-products of fatty acid and carbohydrate metabolism in the liver. An over-abundance of ketones in the bloodstream is seen in a severe metabolic derangement known as diabetic ketoacidosis.

Ketonuria The presence of ketone bodies in the urine.

Latent A dormant state.

LDL A lipoprotein substances (combination of a fat and a protein), which acts as a carrier for cholesterol and fats in the bloodstream.

Lipid Fat.

Lipoatrophy Loss of subcutaneous fat.

Lipohypertrophy An excess of subcutaneous fat, often seen at injection sites.

Lipolysis The breakdown of fat.

Macrovascular Pertaining to large blood vessels.

Microalbuminuria Minute traces of protein in the urine, an early indicator of renal disease in diabetes.

Microvascular Pertaining to small blood vessels.

MODY Mature onset of diabetes in the young.

Monounsaturated A type of fat found in olive oil and rapeseed oil. This type of fat causes the least damage to blood vessels.

Morbidity The incidences of disease or diseases in a population.

Mortality The death rate: the ratio of numbers of deaths to the total population.

Mutation A change in form or characteristic.

Neoplasia New, normally abnormal growth, e.g. a tumour.

Nephropathy A complication related to the kidneys, causing them to leak protein.

Neuroglycopenia Lack of glucose to the nervous system brain, causing symptoms such as blurred vision, headache, slurred speech, confusion, and eventually coma.

Neuropathy A general term denoting functional disturbances and/or pathological changes in the peripheral nervous system.

Pathomechanics A descriptive term for abnormalities in normal processes that lead to some form of tissue injury/destruction.

Phenotype changes resulting in a reaction between a genotype and the environment.

Polyunsaturated A type of fat found in corn and sunflower oil.

Prevalence The proportion of individuals in a population who have a disease.

Proteases An enzyme that breaks down a protein molecule.

Randomized control trial Investigation where at least one group of participants are assigned to a new treatment under scrutiny, whilst a second group receive either a placebo or an established treatment.

Somogyi In diabetes, a rebound phenomenon of reactive hyperglycaemia in response to a preceding period of relative hypoglycaemia that has increased secretion of hyperglycaemic agents (epinephrine, norepinephrine, glucagon, cortisol, and growth hormone).

Systematic review Qualitative research procedure giving a clear audit trail.

Viscosity Stickiness.

Index

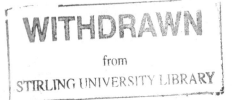